HERBAL and FOLK MEDICINE

of the SOUTH

by Samuel J. Touchstone 1993

Samuel J. Touchstone

TIME

Time changes everything. The song below was a Union song at the beginning of the Civil War. It later became a Southern Ballad near the end of the civil war. The song was sung in the South until the 1940's. If you know the tune to this song, you are old.

THE BOYS IN BLUE

There was an old man,
And he was bent with age,
He landed in this village
After dust was laid.
His voice was meek and low.
Is this the express office, sir?
I'm looking for my son.
They tell me that the train was due
This place at half past one.
O, you have made a sad mistake,
This is an express office, sir,
And not a train depot.
But you don't understand me, sir,(or: The old man shook his head.)
He's not coming as a passenger,
He's coming to me dead.
He's broken his dear mother's heart,
Likewise mine's broken, too.
I told his that he'd come back dead
When he joined the boys in blue.

*****

HERBAL and FOLK MEDICINE of LOUISIANA and the SOUTH

by Samuel J. Touchstone

PB- ISBN: 0-914917-13-7

HERBAL and FOLK MEDICINE of LOUISIANA and the SOUTH

By: Samuel J. Touchstone

publisher.

FOLK-LIFE BOOKS
P.O. Box 128
Princeton, LA 71067

Printed in the United States of America
By:

Century Graphics Corporation
1013 Mcdermott Road
Metaire, LA 70001-6097

① 2 3 4 5

I dedicate this book to my children

and

the old timers

SPECIAL ACKNOWLEDGMENTS

I owe special thanks to many people. First, to my parents who started collecting and recording herbal and folk medicine cures long before I came into this world. Second, to the old timers who shared their most secret cures and treatments with me. Most of these old timers have long since departed this world but their folk medicine lives on.

TABLE OF CONTENTS

The author is or was a member of:

ARK-LA-TEX Gem and Mineral Society, Inc
Bossier Parish Restoration Foundation
North Louisiana Historical Association
The Folk Life Society of Louisiana
Red River Parish Heritage Society

Also Listed in North Louisiana Folk Crafts

The author has lectured on Louisiana Folk Life, herbal and folk medicine and local history to many groups. Several articles have been published in the North Louisiana Historical Journal.

He is also the author of:

Herbal and Folk Medicine of Louisiana & Adjacent States
Folk-Life Series, Vol 1
History of Bossier Parish
Jessie J. Touchstone Family genealogical book

PREFACE

There is not a precise record in existence to determine when herbal remedies were first used. There are Biblical records and records of the Asian Region that indicate the widespread use of herbal medicines since recorded history. The is evidence that the Indians practiced medicine since time unknown in the South. Later, trappers, farmers, housewives and traveling herbal healers used their own home remedies to treat nearly every major malady or minor complaint. By using herbs, simple kitchen product, common fruits and vegetables and other natural ingredients along with wild fruits and herbs, many folk remedies were concocted.

Many of these folk medicine cures continue to be used today and are now of great interest to modern medical researchers. Some of these home cures are far more dangerous than the complaint being treated. Therefore, I strongly advise anyone against trying any of the cures. Should you do so, it is at your risk. Bear in mind that many of these herbal cures do work and some may be more effective than modern medicine

I have many years in active herbal use, the gathering, curing and preparation of herbal cures. I have recorded the herbal information as I have found it was used. The same herbal cures are used all over the South with slight variations. I hope you will use this text as a guide to further the study and recording of herbal and folk medicine.

The book is a record of herbal medicine and is not a DOCTORS BOOK.

FACTS YOU SHOULD KNOW

Herbal and folk medicine cannot be called an exact science. There are many variables such as strength of a herb, strength of dosage, method of preparation, green or dry herb, that will affect the end results of a given herbal treatment. Also, the age, weight, sex and general health will determine the dosage required for a given result.

The medical terms, emetic, diuretic etc. are given for you information as the nearest medical description of the use of a herb by herbal folks. Some of them may not be as accurate as one would desire, but these are as near the proper description as could be determined to give you a general idea as to what the modern medical use would be.

While reading this book, you may get the impression that the earlier folks before you were a bunch of "sicklings." That is far from true. This book gives you a record of the treatments used over a long period and for many people. A given family may not use herbs, other than tonics, once or twice a year. Members of a family having bowel problems would be given a herbal laxative when required.

Herbal medicine was preventive in nature. The diet of the times was lacking in many minerals and vitamins needed for good health. The folks over time learned that certain herbs taken regularly would make them feel and look better. They did not know at that time that the minerals and vitamins in the herbs was causing the effect.

Herbal medicine is just a country drug store. You would no more go into a drug store and start taking random bottles of medicine off the shelf to treat yourself without knowing what the medicine was made to treat.. Likewise, you would not go into the woods and start gathering herbs to take. You must know what they are used to treat or you are in big trouble. You must also know for sure that the herb is what you think it is. There are many look-a-likes in the herbs. There are many herbal stores where you can purchase the herbs you want. Some of the companies are listed in the back of this book. This would be a fairly safe way to obtain the herbs and much easier. Gathering herbs in the wild is quite a chore.

Many years ago, I would hear the old folks saying that "Mr. Smiths snake root & etc. doesn't work as well as Mr. Jones." This was true as herbs gathered on one hill could be different on one side of the hill than the other. The reason being that the soil on one side of the hill may not have the mineral in the soil that has the healing power.

The old timers soon learned who had good herbs. This also applies to the flat lands. An other example to make the point, the flavor of cornmeal grown in different types of soil will taste quite different. Blackland has the best corn flavor.

The only experiences many of you have had with herbs was from watching TV or the movies. A man get shot or injured. A Indian just happens to come by. He looks at the man and runs out in the woods. Very shortly here he comes back with a handful of some type of green leaves or something. He either places it on the wound or makes a brew. The man get us and lives. It don't happen this way. Very seldom will you find the herb near when you need one. Also, most herbal brews or treatments are very slow, sometimes taking days to work. There are some herbs that work instantly, in no uncertain terms.

Faith or strong belief seems to be a great factor in the use of some herbs. I have seen people that looked like "death warmed over" or on "deaths door" be given a herbal brew that did not have any minerals or elements that would cure their ailment. Low and behoo, in a few days they would be up and about. I have seen people who were treated by the "laying on of the hands" show remarkable improvement. They claim it was the "Divine." I think it was that person's faith that it would help that pulled them through. I have also seen where they "laid on the hands" and the person just died. This they said just wasn't god's will." There were many ailments where "laying on the hands," herbs, or any other treatment would help. They would just up and die on you. Each family, through trial and error, would develop a family medical history of each member over the years. This would enable them to determine which herb or herbs, size of dosage, strength and other factors to consider for a given complaint.

The methods of used for some of the herbs in this text were not given because of the many variables. One member of a family would be given the herb as a decoction, another member as a tonic and still a third member as either a salve or poultice or a given complaint.

The "Preparing Herbs" and "Glossary" section should be read and studied before continuing with the remainder of the text so that you will be able to better understand the actual complaints the herbal people were trying to treat.

Many herbal advocates made corn shuck tea, corn silk tea, oat straw tea and even sulphur and molasses tea. It is very difficult to determine just what the teas were given to a person to treat. Some of the herbal users said they were for the kidneys, others said they were for the blood and still some of the people said the teas were given "just because they needed it." Pine straw tea was given for several complaints.

The herbal and folk medicine "cures" were the most common ones used in Louisiana and the South. This is because of the information was obtained from people who had moved into this area from other states years back, bringing their "cures" with them. Some herbs were rarely used and then in a very small area of the state. Their accurate use could not be determined, so they were omitted.

The rural herbal users would not give up on an ailment; they would keep giving anything and everything. Sometimes they would hit on a cure, and other times there was an unscheduled funeral.

The herbal users in sugar cane areas claimed that the "Yellers" (jaundice) was cured by the person chewing large quantities of sugar cane until the "yellers" "went in."

Powdered rice or lint from "under the bed" was used by a small number of herbal users to stop bleeding. Two cups of raw "gobbler peas" (peanuts) were used to "grease" a "stopped up belly" so the "hocky could slide out." One old man claimed that snake root would "cure" snakebite because his dog ran out and ate snake root every time the dog was bitten by a snake. I would not advise you to try this one.

Due to the very limited knowledge or use of the above "cures" by herbal healers, they are listed for your information and further investigation.

Many of the very old rural herbal users said that many of the herbs they used were obtained from the "root man." The most reliable information on the "root man" was that he went from place to place selling and trading for local herbs. This would allow herbal users to obtain herbs that did not grow in their locale. This may account for some of the herbs used by the rural folks that are not known to grow in their area.

Many of the herbal users said they would buy herbs from the "root man" when they went to the "big store" about twice a year. These root peddlers would part their buck board wagons along the roads near the town. The folks from way back would trade farm goods, etc., or other herbs for the ones they needed.

There were also peddlers who went out in the back woods in larger covered wagons selling everything from pot and pans to herbs. They would barter, trade or what have you for anything they could use or sell elsewhere.

Historical accounts of the herbal trade could not be located. Maybe because the peddlers were selling everything from collard greens to fatback along with the herbs.

The history of herbal and folk medicine would not be compete without giving some information on the "Watkins Peddlers." A person would have had to live in a shell if he or she had not heard of Watkins products. The Watkins peddlers started the beginning of the end to herbal medicine in most areas. They sold about fifty different kinds of folk medicine all of which were equal to or better than any other kind of medicine to be had at that time. The Watkins peddlers went from house to house in a buck-board wagon or walked with their case of "cures" and other household items. They filled a need in the rural areas and supplied the news and gossip from other regions of the state. Many of the rural folks paid for the medicine they purchased with farm produce. There were other peddlers with other brands, but Watkins was by far the best known and most used.

Some of the folk medicine treatments were simple and said to be effective. What we know as Dyspepsia today was treated by simple method of slapping the abdomen or "bowels" with the palm of the hand for fifteen minutes in the morning, fifteen minutes at noon, and ten minutes in the evening before retiring. They claimed this is excellent for chronic indigestion. Rubbing and kneading is a very old folks medical treatment. They would also feed people with dyspepsia complaints mashed egg yolks and potatoes with soda biscuits.

COLLOQUIAL: CURE OR TREATMENT

When collecting and recording herbal and folk medicine from rural areas, you will find that every plant or concoction given to you will be called a "cure." Some of the herbal or chemical mixtures will be called a "sure Cure." The word "cure" has several meanings among the herbal users. The folk medicine mixture of sulphur and hog grease smeared on the "itch" was called a "sure fire Cure." This meant that the scratching and the itching would be eliminated until they caught the "itch" again. I don't know why "fire" was added to some cures and not to others.

"Cure" meant to the herbal users what today would be called a treatment. If pain and other discomforts from a given ailment stopped when given, a herbal mixture would be called a "cure," although at times it did nothing for the ailment.

The rural folks would continue giving herbal "cures" to a person "sick unto death" (fatal illness) knowing full well that the person would die.

Seneca and button head snake root was given for the flu or pneumonia. This increased the chance of survival tenfold. Would you call this a "cure" or treatment? It is just a matter of semantics.

In many cases, the herbal user would just say, "(whatever it happened to be) will bring a boil to a head" or "this will stop bleeding," without calling it a "cure" or "treatment."

A few select questions will determine what the herbal user expects of a given herb or concoction. Remember that a concoction and a decoction are not the same.

To further complicate things, some herbal folks used the word "kill" to describe what a herb would do: for example, this herb will kill itch, or this herb will kill TB. Wonder how many times they would admit a herb killed the patient!

DOCTOR OR HERBS

This book is in no way intended to sway you to replace your doctor with herbs and folk medicine. This would be a foolish and dangerous course to follow. Many years back when herbal and folk medicine was in its hay day, doctors were in short supply and their qualifications were in question. Many of the people were just not able to pay a doctor's fee. Also, a good many rural doctors darn near starved trying to live on a the chickens used to pay his fee. Most of the herbal medicine was preventive in nature. They were in fact, supplying their bodies with natural vitamins and minerals which in itself would prevent many illnesses. The very nature of their daily food intake would aid in good health. This is not to way that herbs did not cure or "doctor" anyone as herbs were used many times to cure or aid in the recovery of their "sick folks."

Herbal and folk medicine is returning to use in leaps and bounds at present time. Now, the medical and scientific fields are studying the value of herbs in medicine. They have discovered many chemicals or minerals in herbal plants to prolong life or cure some of the fatal illnesses.

The medical research groups have discovered some of the chemicals in the herbs thought not to be of value were, in fact, used as a buffer or catalyst to the active chemical used for treatment. These buffers or catalyst eliminated the side effects which occur when used man-made chemicals for the same treatment.

This country will require years of study to reach the level other countries have reached in the use of herbs in medicine.

MEDICAL HERBAL TEAS

Some herbs are not safe to ingest or use on the body. Many herbs are perilous to your health, body, limb and soul. I would advise anyone wishing to use herbs to learn about them one at a time and also to learn to use one at a time. Read up on herbs, study them, and talk to people who are already versed in herbal use. Know the herbs you wish to use or leave them alone.

Some herbs have a long record of folk medicine use and appear to be non-toxic, yet they are listed as dangerous for certain internal and external use by some government departments. Some of these warnings may be true and you should seriously investigate them. There are so many safe and valuable herbs and food herbs, so why use herbs that may be dangerous to the central nervous system, or for any other part of the body?

The dose for any given person must be determined by several factors, such as weight, age, general health and other intangible factors. Use half doses or less for children. Take a small amount of the herb and experiment on the person for possible allergic reactions before giving a full dose.

Herbal medicine, whether infusions or decoctions, work show and usually take three day to work. For acute health problems, drink only half a cup three times a day, one half hour before meals. Should the health problem disappear, discontinue taking the tea. If you do not see any change in three days, change the treatment.

Don't be discouraged if the person feels "awful" after an hour or so during the first day or so. Many herbs work slowly before starting to normalize the body, detoxify and cause the body to "blow" out the waste and sometimes, I mean it really blows. Ginger tea and cinnamon sticks are both extremely detoxifying but slow to act. Give any tea a chance to work. There is not one tea that works for everyone; therefore, you will have to experiment with different herbs.

Here is a fairly safe list of herbs that rural folks used when learning to make teas and decoctions. They learned by taste how strong to make tea.

FLOWERS:	Clover and mullein
LEAVES:	Sage, red raspberry, catnip, blackberry, spearmint and peppermint
BERRIES:	Blackberries, blueberry and raspberry
SEEDS:	Anise, caraway, celery, dill and fennel
BARK:	Ginger

One may wish to mix combinations of the above to see what taste one can develop.

To avoid confusion, I will modify the average three days for some herbs to work. The results of some herbs are very fast. The action of external herbs starts on contact in most cases.

There is nothing mysterious or mystic about herbal teas. When you drink a cup of coffee, hot or cold, even a glass of warm mild, you are using herbal or folk medicine teas. Tonics and teas are about the same, other than the tonic is made to be much stronger and for a given complaint. Teas are said to taste good. Folk medicine users say "the worse the taste of the tonic, the better the cure." I will assure you that it takes a lot of effort to down some of the tonics.

The information given on herbal tea is for your information, and in no way or form should you use them without first talking with your doctor or a friend who does use the teas.

This book is a history of the use of herbal and folk medicine as the folks told me or taken from old family records. This does not tell you that it is safe to use any herb or folk medicine.

MIDWIVES AND GRANNY WOMEN

"Midwives" is not an accurate description of the ladies of country medicine. When doctors were scarce, and their skill were suspect and not reliable, midwives were used. Most modern information sources lead people to believe that midwives spent their lives delivering babies. This is just not true before the 1940's. (There were some exceptions in some regions) A large portion of their "healing" time was treating the ill and accidental injuries (some injuries were not so accidental) such as cuts, bruises, broken bones, bleeding, bites, stings and gunshot wounds. The other treatments were for boils, hives and any other medical complaint. Delivering babies was more or less a sideline when the total time spent treating the rural folks is considered. They also was expected to "sit with the dying or dead." They were the most respected folks in the region. They never received much money, but they sure had plenty to eat well with all the foodstuff given for their services. It constist mostly of chicken, "taters" and other farm produce.

These ladies were called "Granny" Jones, Smith, etc. Some called the ladies "Aunt Sara, Beth, etc. Each community had their own "Granny" or Aunt." These people would just say, "Go get Granny" as everyone knew who the Granny was for their community.

Bragging was also a weakness of the backwoods folks. For instance, should their local Granny not be available and another Granny from some other community was needed, family members would brag about their Mary Lue being so sick that a Granny from way "up yonder" was "fetched" to save her life.

"Grannies" were paid very little or nothing for their work although some of the folks would bring different roots and herbs for her to use. This was really for their benefit, not the "Grannies." Some folks paid her well in money or goods. Others thought it was her "job" to treat them, so they didn't owe her "nar a thang."

Around 1940, the government did train many women to be midwives and midwives only. Their job was to deliver babies in the rural areas.

RELIGION IN MEDICINE

Religion for the purpose of this book means "a belief binding the spiritual nature of man to a supernatural being and those things added by mankind to suit his own ideas and power to control the masses," so this refers to no religion or cult in general.

The art of healing by medicine and doctors has been strongly resisted by religious leaders since recorded history. They believe that healing was their field solely and others entering this field would weaken their hold and control of the masses. Some religions now have their own hospitals to assure that their religious dogma is not violated.

Some people believed that reading Ezekiel, 16th Chapter, 6th Verse, bleeding would be stopped. By the time they got their Bible and read the verse several times, the bleeding probably would have stopped of its own accord due to clotting. This is something you can decide for yourself. The verse reads as following: "And when I passed by thee, and saw thee polluted in thine own blood, I said unto thee when thou waste in thy blood, live, yea, I said unto thee when thee waste in thy blood, live." I still say you had better start applying the known blood stopping procedure, for external bleeding.

Some diseases went into remission, either temporarily or permanently after receiving the service of a memb er of the Deity.. This cannot be explained in any way, so this just might be the work of the Divine -- who knows? I still believe the faith the person, with the illness made the body heal itself. I still say if it works, go for it.

Religion cannot be discounted in the healing process, good or bad. The "laying of the hands" and other rites administered by a servant of the Deity to the ill have in some cases resulted in the recovery of the person. The reason was very likely that they were able to raise the level of faith, or the will to recover, in the ill person. This form of psychology could possibly activate the body's own defenses which start producing anti-bodies to cast out or destroy the cause of the illness. Should the person die, they would fall back on the cliche, "It was the will of God."

The religious record is scored zero in cases where vital organs of the body were already damaged and had ceased functioning. Many others claims of healing were not the rites, but the delayed action of medication and treatment given by doctors at an earlier time. Many others receiving the rites did not even have the disease or complaint they believed they had, which established a false credit.

Some men of the cloth relied on both religion and herbal healing. They were always in demand and accepted. Now the people could fulfill their religious beliefs and get medical help without being ostracized by peers or suffering the wrath of the fanatics in the area.

People of faith should get the rites of their belief as soon as they determine they have an illness that could be fatal. It may work and one has nothing to lose by accepting them.

The fire and brimstone preachers of the backwoods were rabid with fanatic beliefs, and more or less developed their own idea of what religion should be. They would prevent their members from seeking medical help by threatening them with fire and brimstone and damnation. Should the father of the household be the religious fanatic, the kids or wife would surely die before he would give in to medical help. But should the mother be the fanatic, at some point the father would overrule her as she had no power as the belief was that her purpose was to bear and raise children, wait on the family: in fact, she was more or less considered just another piece of property.

Other religious groups would surround the person who was ill or afflicted with some malady. They would kick, beat or shove the person. Their belief was that they would beat or run the devil out of the person so they would get well. Sometimes this sadistic rite would greatly harm or injure the person.

A lady named Jones in Massachusetts was hanged in 1640 because she cured people with roots and herbs. They said this as proof she possessed the diabolical powers invested in witches. Even taking a bath was at one time called the work of the devil. Blood transfusions were condemned by; many as blasphemy and going against the will of God. When religious leaders are confronted with this past belief, they say "That was the dark ages." Even today many people let members of their family die trying to pray them well when one or more trips to a doctor could have saved their lives. Several laws were passed to protect the young and helpless. Seldom are these laws enforced and then with only a token slap on the wrist. Far too many cases of this nature never come to the attention of the public so action can be taken. They are overlooked, veiled or just plain forgotten.

Most all religions today support and encourage medical help. The information given here is not an expression of my own views, either pro or con. These values were given in order that one may understand that is difficult to separate medical treatment from religious beliefs in most illnesses.

Who knows, a hundred years from now they may say,

"They were in the dark ages."

SUPERSTITION AND FOLK MEDICINE

Superstition is a belief founded on irrational feelings, especially of fear and marked by credulity. The superstitious folks will never believe otherwise than that their belief is true.

The following is a few of the rural folk medicine beliefs.

A screech own calling from your rooftop is a "sure fire" sign of death for one of your loved ones.

A "lighten-ing bug" (firefly) in the house at night, meant a member of the house would be gone before the next sundown.

A person could blow the fire out of a burn, if he never way his father.

Turning your shoes upside-down at night would cure sore feet.

A black cat's tail could remove a stye.

Wrapping a string around the little toe and standing in fresh cow manure could cure foot itch.

Pulling a nail out of a foot and spitting on it, then throwing the nail over your shoulder would prevent lock-jaw.

Putting scissors with the points up on the neck could stop nosebleed.

Carrying a buckeye in your pocket would prevent illness.

Placing an ax under the bed would cut pain.

There are too many superstitious wart cures to list, one being, "steal the neighbor's dirty dish rag, wipe the warts and carry the dish rag back." The folks with faith could and did conjure warts off, so this may not belong under superstition. While trying to disprove conjuring, research has proven conjuring is a true fact.

"Stye! Stye, leave my eye and catch the next one that comes by." Did you ever use that one when you were a kid?

HERBAL AND FOLK MEDICINE FOLKLORE
The No No's of Folk Medicine

The human ran has entertained their egos by cruel jokes and tricks on the lame, disfigured and those who mental and educational level were in serious doubt compared to what would be considered normal in a given time and place.

Three joke type folk-medicine cures that are passed on to the unknowing public by various forms of communications are the cures using manure. Maybe it is shock treatment or just to get your attention. The three are: making sheep pill tea for hives; cow manure or cow chip tea for sore throat; and smearing black chicken manure on the lips to stop hot pepper from burning. Other joke cures passed on were some that would burn hell out of the user.

Before the 1940's, barn raisings, house raisings, log rollings and chimney "dobbin' " were a common affair. At rest periods at these gatherings, the men would gather in a group to discuss this and that. I remember at several different get-together when some poor soul would ask about a cure for some ailment and these men would give him one of the joke manure cures. These men would snicker and laugh with glee when the man left to try the cure on some member of his family. He probably passed it on to some other people who used it not knowing it was a joke cure. This is how it could have become known as a real cure. Someone who could write recorded them, and at some later date people assumed they were for real.

You did not dare inform the man that the manure cure was a joke, for he would surely go and wipe out whomever gave it to him. Your only hope was to convince him that you had a better cure for that ailment.

Green cow manure (fresh and warm) was used on sprains and other injuries, where the skin was not broken, for temporary relief from pain or swelling, and then only when they were too far from a house. I never used this method, so I don't know if it works or not.

Some Indians and farmers or hunters would stand in piles of warm manure for temporary relief from frostbite.

A common practice to remove mosquitoes from the house was to take a bucket. Punch holes near the bottom and add a couple inches of dirt, then fill the bucket with dry cow-chips. They would then light it and put some green leaves over the top of the cow-chips so it would smother burn and smoke. This would run everybody out of the house including the mosquitoes.

For years urine was collected from convents and sold to chemical firms so they could recover certain hormones from the urine for use in treating certain women ailments. This was before they learned to make hormones.

People put urine on nettle stings to relieve the pain. The above methods are the only ways I know that excreta was a part of folk-medicine, and I wouldn't swear by them.

Did you ever wonder why all some people remember about herbal and folk medicine is "dung" cures and "sassafras" tea? Of the hundreds of herbs and chemicals used in folk medicine, one would believe they would remember more than these two. When someone tells you about an excreta cure, ask them if they have used it. Ask them how they prepared it and what did they use it to cure.

HAPPINESS IN THE FOLK MEDICINE COUNTRY

Happiness today means having a big car, fine home and all the better things in life. At an earlier time in the rural life, happiness had an altogether different meaning. All their family being well and food to eat was happiness to its greatest in the rural backwoods. The following was happiness:

1. The neighbor's wife dies instead of yours.
2. The cow gave half a gallon more milk today.
3. The ice storm broke the limbs on the shade oak instead of your pear tree.
4. There were more potatoes in each hill than last year.
5. The barn burned instead of your house.
6. The chickens lay three more eggs today.
7. One of your three daughters died instead of your only son. (Three sons and one daughter likewise.)
8. Your Uncle's family was too sick to visit you this Christmas.
9. Your child broke his arm instead of his or her leg.
10. You made it to the bean pot before the others.

So you see, happiness had an altogether different meaning to the people in the rural backwoods of yesterday than what people of today call being happy. The rural folk's view was that it could have been worse.

These people did not have welfare, social security, free cheese, food stamps, free medical care, and other government handouts. Their survival depended on their own "grim, grit and guts" to have food, shelter, and good health. They spent most of their time raising, finding, gathering, and storing food for themselves, the farm animals, and some extra for the hard times when the crops were poor. Anything less than worse would give them reason to be happy.

COLLOQUIAL MEASUREMENTS

Scales for weighing herbs and what have you just did not exist in rural or frontier sections during the heydays of herbal use. At a later period, cotton scales, both bale and picking size, were available most everywhere but they could not be used for herbal measurements. Any book where herbal measurements are given in pounds, ounces, grams and grains, should be suspect. They are either modern or copied from some early period doctor book. Listed below are some of the most common units of measure used during the prime herbal period.

SMIDGEN	HEAPING-SPOON	QUART
PINCH	CUP	GALLON
DROP	HANDFUL	SYRUP BUCKET
DASH	DOUBLE-HANDFUL	PECK
THIMBLE	DIPPER	BUSHEL
SPOONFUL	PINT	HALF-BUSHEL
MITE	"Toe-sack" (Tote-sack, burlap, hemp or croaker sack)	

Any herbal cure where the amount to be used is given as a smidgen, pinch or drop, you had better heed. It is nearly always a sure warning that the herb used is dangerous or poisonous. Many variances occur in preparing herbal brews and where larger doses than a cup is given, a cup more or less won't alter the remedy.

The medical folklore units of measure may seem quite crude. You can rest assured that the people of that period were very accurate, and should you be inclined to shortchange them, they would let you know in no uncertain terms.

Many of the containers of that time were manufactured with sub-measurements impressed on them, such as ¼ cup, ½ cup on glass containers. A gallon container would have, 1-qt, 2-qt, 3-qt, lines impressed on it.

PATENT MEDICINE or CHEMICALS

Many patent medicines and chemicals were available and used with or in conjunction with herbal remedies, dating back before the Civil War period. Many more chemical preparation were added through the years. By 1940, there were hundreds of them. Most were worthless or dangerous.

Many of these drugs were deadly poison with little or no warning on the container. Some of the poisons came in bottles with little bumps all over the bottle to warn you that it was poisonous. Most homes had poor lighting, so when they felt the bumps on the bottle, they knew it was poison and would not take it by mistake. Most of the more dangerous chemicals were only used by doctors in preparing their chemical cures. Many patients were sent to the "great beyond" after using some of these doctor's chemical remedies. Doctors or drugs were not regulated at that time.

The following page is a general list of the types of chemicals and patent medicines available.

- ALCOHOL
- AMMONIA
- ARSENIC
- ASAFETIDA
- BAKING SODA
- ROUGH ON RATS
- BORIC ACID
- BROMO-QUININE
- CAMPHOR
- CARBOLIC ACID
- COPPERS (Copperas)
- ETHER
- FOWLERS SOLUTION
- GLYCERIN
- IODINE
- IPECA
- PAREGORIC (Opium)
- BLUE STONE (Blue Vitriol)
- PARISH GREEN
- SULPHUR
- QUICK LIME
- TAR (CREOSOTE)
- WHITE ARSENIC
- VASELINE
- QUININE
- VICKS SALVE
- SALT PETER (Saltpetre, nitrate of potash)
- LAUDANUM (Opium Morphine)
- BLACK LEAF 40 (tobacco extract)
- BLUME ASS (Blue mass) (mercury)
- NUX VOMICA (Strychnine)
- BLACK OXIDE (For flies)

Some of the above names are colloquial terms. The folk medicinal use of some of this list will be covered later in this book.

CONCOCTIONS IN FOLK MEDICINE

As the years of herbal use slowly passed, chemical and patent medicines quickly, but surely took the lead in popular use in the backwoods folk medicine. "Blume Ass" (Blue mass), black draugth, and epsom salts which replaced alion strychnine, belladonna and cascara pills, also replacing herbs in the treatment of "costiveness" (constipation). Most often, in the spring, each member of a family would be given one of these purgatives to clean out the system, more or less, as constipation was not a problem. The sanitary conditions the backwoods people lived with would assure they experienced the "runs" in one of the several degrees, quite often, therefore eliminating constipation. A few of the old folks continued to use herbs for constipation as they were afraid of them "furrin" cures.

Hog lard or grease was the base for external concoctions, although "taller" (tallow), turpentine, vaseline and "kol-awl" (kerosene) were used in common remedies. Water was used as a base with epsom salts. The dosage was listed on the patent medicines, but many of the bad woods people added more to the dosage, as their belief was that if a little bit was good, then a "hol- lot" was better. Others could not read, so if the "main Man" at the "big store" didn't tell them how to use the medicine, they guessed. Sometimes they would ask a neighbor how much of a given medicine their family used for a "round" (dosage), then he or she would say "Why, that's the way we use it," not indicating that he or she could not read.

The conconctions most commonly used will be given in this book. The variations are so numerous that it would require a book to cover all of them. The variations in the contents of the concoctions from family to family would not change the outcome of the treatment to the extent that it would require a separate listing.

Alcohol used by the folk medicine people was a high proof spirits. It was used to make extract of herbs and to wash down a patient with high fever. Alcohol was used to clean cuts and wounds.

Ammonia was used as chest rub, for stings (insects or plants), and to rub down sprains, man or beast.

Asafetida was used as a nervine stimulant, powerful anti-spasmodic, expectorant and carminative. It was used as a treatment for infantile pneumonia and flatulent colic. Asafetida was overrated in folk medicine as a cure A few of the backwoods folks made beads from Job's tears (coix lachrymal) and soaked them in asafetida for their children to wear in the wintertime. Others just tied asafetida in a bag around the child' neck. I believe this was more effective in keeping company away than colds.

Baking soda was used to relieve "grease gut" or "heartburn" (indigestion). A teaspoon of soda to a glass of water was the normal dosage. Soda was also used to make foaming tonic drinks. Baking soda was used to draw the "fire" out of the burn, relieve "sour craw", and "gas."

"Blume ass" (blue mass) was used as a purgative. It contains mercury and was a very harsh laxative. Rubbing a penny with blue mass will coat a penny silver bright.

Boric acid was used to clean cuts and wounds.

Quinine was used to treat any complaint to reduce fever. Quinine may raise blood pressure so its use should be controlled.

Camphor was mixed with hog grease or "taller" (tallow) and used as a chest rub. It was also used for sprains and sore joints.

Chloroform was mixed with black cherry extract and used to relieve a cough. Few backwoods folks used chloroform as they had heard "bad omens" about it.

"Coppers" (copperas) was used to build or clean up "bad blood," although they used it for anything else the backwoods folks thought it would help.

Vicks salve was used in folk medicine for any complaint of the chest. They rubbed it on the chest, crammed it into the nose and ate a little of it.

Laudanum (opium morphine) was used for "bad, bad complaints" like TB etc. Some folks did use it for earache. Others put a drop or two in a spoon of syrup to give to their babies to keep them from crying.

The wives slipped "salt peter" (saltpetre, nitrate of potash) in their husband's coffee to slow or stop their sex drive. The military put saltpetre in the food for the same purpose for years before it was stopped by law.

Iodine was used on sores, cuts and wounds to keep them from becoming "proud" (gangrene?). They took a small amount of iodine for "big glands" (goiter?)

Paregoric (opium) was used by the folks just about every time pain was present. It was used for stomachaches, earaches, etc. It was very much misused.

Nux vomica was fed to the chickens to poison hawks should they eat the chickens. The old-timers took a smidgen for "dropsy" and heart complaints. Nux vomica contains strychnine, a deadly poison, so stay clear of it.

Salicylic acid was used to keep their canning from becoming "tainted" (spoiled).

Sulphur and hog grease was used by the folks to kill the itch. It was and still a sure cure.

Turpentine (medicinal) was used on cuts, scratches and bruises. The old folks put a few drops of turpentine on a teaspoon of sugar to take for a cough or cold.

Epsom salts was used as a purgative to really clean out the system, although it was mild in action. Epsom salts was used to soak the feet and hands. It was mixed in ample warm water for a foot or hand bath to ease swelling or other pains. The skin can absorb epsom salts, so too long a period of exposure may result in the "runs." A poultice was made of epsom salts to other parts of the body.

Cream of tartar (potassium bitartrate) may have been of some aid in treating dropsy. The folks claimed it helped any number of complaints, but I believe they just liked the taste. Cream of tartar has an acidulous taste. The old folks would mix water and vinegar to taste, add sugar to taste in a glass. They would then put about a teaspoon of cream of tartar in the glass and stir. A teaspoon of baking soda was then dumped in with a quick stir and they would drink it down fast before it foamed over. Their children would just mix vinegar, water, sugar to taste, add soda and drink as the mother kept the cream of tartar hidden.
Cream of tartar was used for nose bleed and catarrh.

NOTE

This book is a history of folk medicine in the south and must not be used as a doctor's book. This is just a small number of the concoctions prepared and used in rural folk medicine.

ODDS AND ENDS OF FOLK MEDICINE

The following folk medicine treatments are simple and should not require much detail.

Baby powder was made to treat the babies' bottoms by taking dirt form the fire box wall of the dirt chimney. They would powder it fine and tie it up in a bag in order to dust it on The powder was very effective.

Right-handed mothers took the dirt from the left side of the chimney and left-handed mothers took it from the right side. Bear in mind that a left and right handed person may of live in the house at different times. If you ever see an old dirt chimney, look for the chip marks and see for yourself.

A fast way to treat something in a man's eye is to pull a hair out of his upper lip. Try it, the tears will flow flushing the eye.

Bleeding was controlled in several ways, depending on where the person was located when the bleeding started. Near a house, flour was held on the bleeding. Powdered okra was sometimes placed on the bleeding and held with a compress. Some took smut from the smut box of the stove to stop bleeding and sometimes added spider webs with it, if they could find any.

A large percentage of the folks had a mortal obsession about being buried alive. Nearly every family would tell you a tale about how Aunt So & So was most surely buried alive. Granny women would hold a mirror near the nose of the patient and look for moisture. They would also take a hot fire coal or heat a pin very hot and touch it to the patient's skin. If a blister forms, the patient is still alive; if no blister, the patient is buried. The dead were buried in short order, as they didn't want to wait until people could "smell them." Anyway, life was hard and they had to get on with the task of living.

Broken bones were very "bad medicine" in the rural areas. Broken legs or arms were wrapped with "toe-sack" (burlap). A first layer was placed on the leg or arm and then a board was placed on each side. Then they wrapped the leg or arm again. They did little or nothing to straighten the bone, they just left it to fate to heal. Many of the breaks healed crooked and out of shape.

The very knowledgeable grannies would try to straighten the break and make a cast of mud and straw, not unlike the mud and straw used in mud chimneys. I remember seeing one of these cast sometime in the early thirties. I do not know how common the use of mud cast was. I could not find any information in any records of its use. The rural folks would have to carry the member to a "city doctor" with a compound fracture, which was an extended trip. The "city doctor" would either fix it or cut it off. Most times the wound was already well infected, so there was not much the doctor could do.

The old-timers would collect "piss ants" from old pine stumps and make an extract from the ants. They used the extract, according to them, to enable "bloated" folks to "poot" the gas out. This don't make sense as making more gas would not help the problem. Misuse of cures was to be expected, as someone put some of the piss ant extract in the drinking bucket at a dance. The dance ended at a much earlier time than planned.

Bur-goo" or "Burgoo" was a corn porridge much used to keep the "sicks" stomach from "turning over." It was a highly seasoned soup or stew of meats, especially game and vegetables. In fact, it was good eating anytime.

Ginger was added when cooking dry beans to prevent gas. The old folks claimed that ginger or any cookie (syrup cookies) would help you get to sleep, and that milk would retard sleep.

"Bear-grass is common in most areas of the south. It was most used as a binder to bind this and that. Bear-grass is green, although there is some rare red bear-grass near Saline, Louisiana. It was also pulped and used like soap to clean the hands and what have you. A few rural folks claim to have used "bear-grass" in their wash pots. They said, "Just have to battle the clothes a little more."

The mud eaters!! Yes, there were people who ate mud. Some ate red clay, other blue mud, and still other ate the dark gray clay. I do not know the whys or hows of why they ate the mud. It was not very smart to ask one of them why they ate it. The communities did not consider this "normal," so these people were very closed mouthed.

OTHER FACT AND THOUGHTS

In the not too far past, herbs were available only in the local forests and fields, or at least they were obtained from a not too far distance. Now nearly every herb in any form can be obtained from reliable supply houses. You would be very wise to obtain your herbs from these sources as only very knowledgeable herbalists should ever attempt to use herbs from the wild. The "look-a-likes" can send you to the great beyond in short order. Your local library has many books to aid you in identifying herbs, but person to person is still the most reliable method.

A man near Blanchard, Louisiana said the Negro people were still coming to his place to get fresh-green cow manure to make a tea to treat something. Another lady has a letter written just after the turn of the century where a man wrote his wife telling her to use the white from chicken manure to rub on her gums to treat "bad gums." (Pyorrhea?) Did you ever have a person tell you he or she used manure teas? They always tell you that a neighbor or someone else used manure tea to cure some ailment! Now, don't run out and make a batch of manure tea because you will vomit it up before it reaches bottom. Manure teas are dangerous and do not cure or treat any ailment, so leave them be.

Another folk medicine seldom mentioned, although

used quite often, is gelatin. The rural people made gelatin by boiling cowhides, bones and hoofs producing a hard, transparent, tasteless, colloidal protein. This gelatin stock was used as a base for several cures and also to feed the very ill. I do not know where or when they learned this procedure, but you eat the same thing each time you eat jello.

The commercial "Jello" you eat today for dessert is the same gelatin colored and flavored. This gelatin is made in the same manner as the rural folks, only on a much larger volume. Gelatin is a very good food source.

A soup, made with chicken, gelatin and cayenne pepper, was given to treat head colds, chest congestion and several other complaints.

A fumigator was made by the rural folks using cayenne pepper. The dry cayenne pepper was ground into powder and placed on a jar lid. A wire frame was made to hold the lid high enough to place a burning candle under the lid.

They would then close the door to the room while the pepper was doing its work.

Head lice was a problem in many households. They use sassafras oil. I do not know just how they obtained the oil. I believe they just boiled the roots and let it settle, then strained the oil off. It was rubbed into the hair and scalp. Rue was also used to control head lice and other parasites. Rue was used as a ringworm lotion. The rue was prepared by steeping in white vinegar for about a week, sometimes longer. Sometimes a small amount of sulphur was added. The smell of this cure would assure that a person had a day all by their "lonesome."

Sage bunches were hung around the house and porches to repel insects; some of the insects seemed to enjoy sage.

A few of the old-timers claimed that eating quite a few young blackberry shoots "cured" loose teeth. This remains to be seen, as the same folks were muley mouthed.

Even the turnip was used in folk medicine. They were boiled and made into a pulp with a little garlic prepared in the same manner. This pulp was applied to sores, abscesses and rheumatic areas. It seems to have had some merit.

An extract of huckleberry was used to treat burns, scalds, and lesions. The huckleberry season is very short, so I don't believe this cure was used very often. The blueberry is just a commercially improved huckleberry.

Black gunpowder was placed on a wound and set afire to stop bleeding and infections. A hot rod was also used to burn a bad wound or sore for the same purpose. This treatment was very painful so it was used only to save life and limb.

The mulberry was mostly used as a food. In some areas, it was used to treat "sugar" (diabetes) by making a tea from the leaves. At one time the bark from the root was used as a cathartic and to kill tapeworms. The fruit was used to make wine, jams and jelly. The mulberry did not rank very high in herbal use.

Alfalfa contains protein (16%), fat (3%), vitamins C, B_1, B_2, D, E, K, provitamin A; several mineral salts, including potassium, calcium and phosphorus; choline, timentylamine, betaine, alfalfa saponin; an alkaloid, stachydine; a bitter principle; a hormonal substance, coumestrol. The alfalfa is, by its contents, an outstanding herb. The rural herbal users just did not use it very often. The Indians used the seed as an abortifacient and rural folks used alfalfa to increase milk flow in nursing mothers. Herbal users of today should give this herb a second look.

Many herbs were used in combination with one or several other herbs with good results. You better take note also that the mixing of some herbs will result in a completely different result than you expected and not always good.

Some men ate hog testicles, believing it would build up their sex power; others ate brains and eggs to build up their brains. One Grandma said, "Some of the mixings men come up with would puke a "mag-get."

This book is a history of folk medicine and in no way indicates one should try any of them.

DRINKING WATER

The drinking water in the rural areas could be bad for your health and you better think twice before drinking. The water could come from a creek, spring or a shallow well in the path of the run off from the toilet or hog pen. In the summer time, most all the water must be strained to remove the wiggletails before drinking.

Many years back, a Mr. S. T., a Civil War historian, went along with me on one of the interviews in the far backwoods and I do mean far back. The last road to the house was too bad to travel with a truck, so we walked. The weather was very hot, so when we arrived at the house of the interview, Mr. S. T. asked for a drink of water. After asking for the water, I informed him he would have to drink some of the water as they would take a dim view of him after asking for the water. A girl come out of the house with a water bucket and a gourd dipper, and from the teethmarks around the gourd, it looked as if it had been used for about ten years. The only place clean on the dipper was where the teeth marks had cut through the grease and dirt. The girl had sores and blisters all around her mouth and pus seeping out. Mr. S. T. drank out of the dipper next to the handle, trying to avoid where he thought she had drank. She said, "Why, Mr., you are the only person I know who drinks from the dipper from the same place I do."

Upon leaving the house, we saw some member of the house getting water out of a spring in a draw. Up above the draw was the hog pen, cow barn and the outhouse.

The water doesn't seem to harm the rural "folks," but you had better carry your water with you.

HOME POMADE

Even the ladies of the rural areas had a desire to smell fragrant and fresh. This was accomplished by several means, such as eating dried orange peels, putting vanilla extract on their body, fresh cut flowers in their handbag, and some made their own crude pomade. Many more just took along fresh small limbs from the sassafras to chew on to freshen their breath.

They made the pomade by smearing tallow or hog grease over a sheet of glass or a granite pan if glass was not available. They would spread fresh flowers (most time yellow jasmine) over the glass or pan. The ladies would then place the glass or pan in a dark place until the next day. Again the flowers would be replaced with fresh ones and placed back in the dark. The ladies would repeat this process for ten to twenty days, depending on how strong they wished the pomade to be.

The women and girls wiped a small amount of the grease or tallow from the glass or pan and smeared it on their person when going to "Sunday-go-meeting," "a death watch," or some other backwoods social function, such as they were.

Some of the more learned rural women placed the tallow or grease pomade in alcohol to remove the tallow or grease and make a cleaner and much stronger perfume.

Even today "store bought" pomade is sold as "pomade 20, 30, or 50." The number following the pomade indicates the number of times the flowers were changed for that batch. You may make your own pomade by using the above method, crude but effective.

SOFT BREAD

Soft bread is made from corn pulled from the field before it is dry. The people made soft bread when there was no food and they had to eat. Other times, the soft bread was used in medical treatments such as poultices and stomach ailments.

The grating device was a syrup bucket lid with many holes punched in it with a nail. This soft meal was prepared the same as dry ground meal.

For folk medicine, it was made into a mush when used as a poultice and made into a gruel (a semi-liquid food made by boiling meal in water or milk) for stomach complaints with and without herbs.

You should try some soft bread, you will be pleasantly surprised. It is some what sweet.

It was not uncommon for the rural folks to add cayenne pepper, garlic or onions to their regular corn bread to keep the "sniffles" from turning into "new-mooney." Other herbs were sometimes added to their bread to keep them going "til cottn' piken was over." As a "pone" of cornbread was their noon meal while working in the field, they may have put the herbs in it for a better taste. they had to eat the cornbread cold when working in the field.

Most of the meal used in the rural areas was whole corn, stone-ground. They said that "bolted" meal (factory-ground) was bad for the health. (Factory meal is sifted, removing the husks, which is part of the taste.)

HONEY

Honey contains: calcium, potassium, aluminum, sodium, copper, iron, manganese, phosphorus, magnesium, sugars, silica, chlorine, vitamins and other qualities.

Honey has all but disappeared from the daily diet and use as a medical remedy in the present times. Contrary to popular belief, honey never was anything but a sometimes item in the daily rural diet. The major, and most times, only source of honey in the rural areas was from wild bee hives in trees. The recovery of this honey required a good bit of time and energy, so by far the greater part of the honey was retained for use in medical remedies.

The chemical contents of honey varied greatly from place to place. The dark honey has far more minerals than the lighter colored honey. Honey slung from the cones will have its full mineral contents as made by the bees, whereas commercially processed honey will go through a heat process which destroys some of the minerals and vitamins. They may also add an extender.

Uncooked honey may contain botulism organism which is easily digested by adults. According to the Center for Disease Control in Atlanta, children under the age of one year should not eat raw honey as it will cause a terrible diarrhea.

Rural folks dabbed honey on small cuts, scratches and blisters which would aid healing by its ability to destroy bacteria. Honey's affinity to water allows it to draw water from bacterial cells; therefore, causes them to shrivel and die.

Many of the people said that honey and/or honey comb would "cure" hay fever, although not one of them had used this method. The "cure" was to eat a spoonful of honey after each meal and chew honeycomb several times each day during the "hay fever" season. I asked a friend to try this honey treatment and the results were disappointing. This does not mean that it would not work on other people.

All the rural folks at one time or the other had the "dry heaves" (also called "dry pukes" and "dry throw-ups.") "Dry heaves" meant violent vomiting with the ejecting of little matter (vomiturition).

The rural folks mixed a cup of honey to a gallon of warm water as a "cure" for "dry heaves." The person with this ailment would continue drinking this mixture after each ejection until the vomiting ceased.

The old-timers claimed honey would induce sleep. They made a mixture of three or four spoons of apple cider vinegar to about a cup of honey. This mixture was placed in a sealed jar. The dosage was a spoonful before bed time. They also used this mixture for coughs.

Many farmers would eat a couple of spoonfuls of honey so they could ward off fatigue until they finished that last hour of plowing in the late evening.

Honey was used as a base in several herbal ointments.

Honey wine (mead) is made with honey and water placed in a stone crock in the dark and allowed to ferment for about thirty days. Many a wife got tipsy testing to see if the wine was ready. The old-folks say, "Honey wine is good for what ails you."

Many of the rural women said that they mixed honey and egg white to "cure bad skin" on the face. They spread the mixture over the face and let it dry for about one hour before washing it off.

Honey was used to sweeten or flavor some of the bad tasting herbal mixtures.

Honey was also used to regulate the bowels."

HONEY DEW

Honey dew is a sweet, saccharine substance found on the leaves of trees and other plants in small drops like dew. It is most often found on the leaves of the sweet gum, maybe because it is easy to see. It is deposited on the leaves in drops as large as a quarter. It is very sweet and thick like bee honey.

The folks claimed it had many healing properties, maybe because it appeared like magic and they did not know how it happened. Honey dew is a good source of food while in the woods. Honey dew is found mostly on small sweetgums and easy to reach with their tongue. You could make a meal on it, but you sure would have to do an awful lot of licking.

They claim that apple cider vinegar mixed with honey or honey dew and given in the same manner as for "dry heaves" would cure the "gripes." (The gripes is the same as "dry heaves" except the problem is on the other end)

HERBS USED IN THE SOUTH

B	Bark	R	Roots
F	Fruit or Flowers	S	Seeds
L	Leaves	X	Whole Plant
P	Whole Plant, except Roots		

Agrimony	X
Aloe Vera	L
American Centaury	L F
American Mandrake	R
Asparagus	X
Bayberry	B
Bay Tree	L F
Beach	B L
Bellwort	R
Bethroot	R
Bindweed	R
Bitter Weed	P
Blackberry	X
Black Haw	R B F
Blue Flag	R
Boneset	X
Caraway	S
Carrot	R S
Castor Bean	S
Cayenne Pepper	F
Cherry Laurel	X
Chickweed	P
Chicory	L R
Clover, Red	X
Clover, White	X
Clover, Yellow	X
Collards	L
Colt's Foot	L F
Foxglove	L
Fringe Tree	B
Garlic Bulb	Bulb
Golden Rod	P
Gravel Root	R
Hollyhock	P
Horse Mint	X
Horseradish	R
Ice Vine	X
Indian Turnip	X
Indian Pipe	X
Iron Wood	Heart
Jerusalem Oak	X
Jimson Weed	L
Juniper	F
Lavender	P
Lemon	F
Lettuce	L
Lily-of-the-valley	R F
Lizard's Tail	R
Lobelia	F P
Marigold	P
Mayweed	R
Buttonhead Snakeroot	R
Milkweed	R
Milkweed, Butterfly	P
Mistletoe	F
Mullein	L F

Comfrey	X	Mustard	LF
Cotton	R	Nettle, Stinging	L
Cucumber Tree	F	New Jersey Tea	B
Dandelion	X	Oats	P
Deer's Tongue	X	Okra	F S
Devil's Bit	R	Onion	Bulb
Dill	L S	Passion Flower	F
Dogwood	X	Partridge Berry	P
Elder	X	Peach tree	L F
Fennel	X	Peony	R
Fig	F	Persimmon	B F
Pink Root	R	Sneezewort	X
Poison Hemlock	L	Strawberry	X
Poke Weed	R F L	Sumac	P F
Polypody Root	R	Tobacco	L
Pomegranate	B F	Virginia Snake Root	X
Prickly Ash	B	Watercress	P
Pumpkin	S	Water Melon	F
Purslane	X	White Oak	B
Raspberry	X	White Snake Root	R
Rattle Box	S	White Water Lily	R
Rue	P	Wild Cherry	B F
Saffron Crocus	R	Wild-Ginger	B F
Sage	L	Wild Indigo	B
Sassafras	X	Willow, Common	B L
Self Heal	P	Wormwood	X
Senna Snake Root	R	Yarrow	P
Slippery Elm	B	Yellow Jessamine	R
Smartweed	X	Yellow Lady's Slipper	R

Many of these herbs were in common use throughout the South. Some of the herbs are limited in use to a very small locale in different areas. There are many more herbs were not listed because they had little or no use in herbal medicine. Others, I could not find anyone that used them. This does not mean they were not used.

COLLECTING HERBS

All parts of plants contain chemicals, but collect only those parts that you intend to use. Some plants are now very hard to find. By taking part of the leaves or flowers only from each plant, you may save a few of the plants for future use.

Many habitats of the herbal plants have been destroyed. This has forced many herbal users to grow some of the more common herbs. (types easy to grow) There are plenty of herb stores selling seed and sets. You can grow them in pots or in small areas of your yard. Some have beautiful flowers and scent. This would be an asset to your home.

Herbal collectors should be sure the herb they collect is the herb they think it or somebody will be burying your mistake. The victims of your mistake may not be around to complain.

Always collect plants after the dew is off as they will be less likely to mold. Mold is a big problem with collected herbs.

Collect flowers as soon as they have opened completed. Collect leaves when they are fully developed just before the flowers fade. Aromatic herbs are gathered when the plant is in bloom. Collect stalks in the fall. Also, collect twigs in the fall. Gather bark, root and branch bark in the fall or early spring. Collect seeds anytime before they mature to use in treatments.

Gather annuals just before flowering. Gather biannuals after vegetation of the first year is over. Gather perennials either in the spring before vegetation begins or in the fall after vegetation is over.

Many of the rural users did not gather any herbal

plants until they needed them, so they were sometimes left "holding the bag" or "bummed" them from somebody who had collected them.

Collecting herbal roots requires some effort and skill. You should know something about the physical size and length of the herb root when digging, as each different herb varies somewhat. Spade a circle about six to ten inches from the stem of the herb and deep enough to recover all or most of the main root. Turn the circle of dirt out with the plant. Now break the lumps of dirt off carefully in a manner to recover as much of the root as you can. Catch the herb by the stem and shake to dislodge as much of the small bits of soil as you are able to remove without damaging the root. Place the root in a paper bag and label with the full name of the herb. Repeat the above procedure on the other herbal roots you plan to collect on a given trip.

Should you intend to use the herbal roots immediately, wash clean and prepare the herb according to the use required. To dry for future use, dip wash the root and blot dry with paper. Hang the blot dried root or roots under an open-air shed and let them air dry. Herbal roots may be heat dried, but the results may not be suitable. Larger roots are cleaned and sliced into small bits and hung up in a burlap bag to dry. The root will loose some of the juice before it dries in this manner. The whole root method of drying will retain all the juices.

Seneca snake root is heat sensitive; therefore, it should be air dried, ground to a powder and stored in a tight container. Any herb requiring a cold infusion to prepare for use should also be open-air dried.

After drying, all herbal roots should be stored in a dark, dry location.

Drying of the herbal flowers or blooms require more attention during the drying process. Pick the flowers and spread them out on paper in the sun for about thirty minutes. This will reduce the chance of mold. Move the flowers and paper to a dry shade, and turn the flowers over several times the first day and as required until dry. Flowers can be strung on strings and hung to dry in a shade after removing from the sun treatment. After the flowers are dry, they can be stored in paper bags filled loosely with the top of the sack pinned shut.

Single picked herbal leaves are also placed on paper in the sun for about 30 minutes before moving to a dry shed to complete the drying process. Turn the leaves several times a day until dry. Store in the same manner as flowers.

Herbs with small leaves are picked by the whole stem. They are also placed in the sun for thirty minutes, turning on time. They are then hung up by a string under a dry shed until dry. When dry, the leaves are removed from the stems by placing them on a hard flat surface and rolled with a rolling pin or some other round item. Remove and discard the stems. Sack the now crushed leaves for storage.

Some herbs (like clover) have a chemical change upon drying; this you must remember when going from fresh to dry herbs. Some of the chemical and minerals change into some other form and are not now the same herb as when green.

Some herbs cannot be gathered and dried as they will lose all their medicinal value when dried. The strength and value of a few herbs will change from location to location. This could be from one hill to the next and etc. The areas called red land may give a problem.

PREPARING HERBS OR MEDICATION

Infusions

Infusions are better known as steeping, not unlike making a pot of tea and most likely called "teas." Leaves and flowers and, in some cases, whole plants are soluble in liquids, usually water. There are hot and cold infusions. Experience or passed-on information will determine which plant is for hot or cold water.

The characteristic flavor of herbal tea comes from the high tannin contents of the leaves. Fresh leaves may not have an aroma. The aroma is formed during the drying or fermentation of the leaves.

Cold infusions are made by soaking in cold water or milk for several hours. The milk may "blue john" on you. Milk is used to increase the healing ability of herb poultices and compresses.

For hot infusions, take the plant or roots and place them in a pot. Pour boiling water over them and place them where it will stay hot. After a few minutes, drain off the liquid. Add something to make it more agreeable to the taste, like milk or sugar. Infusions do not keep well, so they are made normally for immediate use.

Use one teaspoon of herb to each cup of boiling water for weak teas. Leaves, flowers and berries should be slightly mashed to help reduce their aromatic oils. Add less water for strong teas. Dry herbs require less than fresh to make the same strength tea. Herbal teas made with bruised seeds such as fennel, anise, caraway, coriander or cumin may be served piping hot to improve both taste and stomach-easing qualities.

One way to preserve an infusion is to make it three

times as strong as the ordinary infusion. Add one part spirits to every three parts infusion. To use, dilute with three parts water to one of the infusion.

DECOCTIONS

Decoctions are not secret ways to prepare medicines; every time you boil vegetables to eat, you are making a decoction. Should you strain off the liquid, you would have a decoction exactly like the ones used in herbal medicines.

Herbal plants were prepared in this manner when the soluble ingredients will not yield in cold or boiling hot water as used in preparing infusions. Place the herb in the proper type of container and simmer in almost boiling water for half an hour or more. You are really making a soup stock from tough herbs.

Decoctions should always be strained while hot, so the drugs which separate on cooling may be mixed again, if needed, with the fluid by shaking the remedy.

Cook in ceramic, glass, earthenware pots, and as most people use, enameled pots. Astringent plants will absorb the metals from other types of pots. You can preserve decoctions in the same manner you preserve infusions. Do not use aluminum pan.

Examples of plants to be decocted: Barley, elm bark, flaxseed, oak bark, cherry bark and some gum resins.

The strength of decoctions is determined by the amount of herbs to water used and also how hot and long you cook them. Add sugar to the strained juice and continue to boil until most of the liquid is gone to make a very strong brew. Place in bottle and add a little glycerin so it will keep.

TINCTURES

To make a tincture, take the herbs to be used and beat them to a pulp. Add two cups of water and two cups of ethyl alcohol or spirits for every cup of herb. Pour into a large bottle and set in a dark cool place for about two weeks. Drain off the liquid from the bottle, being careful not to stir up the drugs on the bottom. Place the drained off liquid in a clean bottle and add a teaspoon of glycerin for each cup of herb. Tinctures may also be made with wine and brandy. Apple cider is used in some special preparations.

Another way to make tinctures is to put the herbs in a bag and suspend them so alcohol or spirits can drip through the bag and be caught in a container below about the same way coffee is may by dripping.

Tinctures are very concentrated extracts of herbs preserved in alcohol, so very little is required for a dose. From five to fifteen drops at a time is an average dose.

When using hot or cold herbal teas for external use in compresses, foot baths and other uses, add a few drops of tincture for additional remedial action.

Compound tinctures may be made by mixing several herbal tinctures together. Make each type of herbal tincture separate and mix them.

PLASTERS

Plasters are semisolid medicines spread on a cloth or some other flexible medium for application on the external parts of the body. They are named by whatever herb or herbs you use. Plaster of Paris was said to be used where the injured part should not move: i.e., fractured bones. I would not use plaster of Paris over a plaster. This would do more harm than good.

POULTICES

Poultices are made of soft substances, such as ground barks, cornmeal, bread and milk, etc. They are usually applied hot. A poultice is a method of applying moist heat. Poulticies are used to relieve pain and bring blood to the surface. This aids in relieving congestion. They also bring pus to the surface.

POWDERS

Powders is any substance ground very fine and is used in the dry state.

FORMENTATIONS

Fomentations are applied locally. To make, place the herbs to be used in two bags large enough to cover the place to be treated. Steep, wring the liquid out of the bags and apply hot. Use the bags alternately and keep them hot.

SALVES

Salves are about eighty percent vehicle, like lard, tallow or vaseline. The rest is made of whatever herb or drug you need to use.

More herbs are used in the form of a salve than any other method. This is because it is more easy to use, store, and seems to keep its strength longer. As lard was used as the vehicle in nearly all salve, they could convert it for internal use also.

There were so many ways the rural herbal folks prepared herbs for medicinal use, one could never know for sure what method was used. The herbal users prepared the herbs in a manner that they knew would work and could care less what the method was called.

HERBS AND HOW THEY WERE USED

ALOE VERA (Aloe Vulgars & etc.)

Aloe vera will be found as a house plant in many of the home in the South. They were sometimes handed down from mother to daughter, etc. Others took part of a plant and re-potted it.

The juice from the leaves or stalks were used as a fast and ready treatment for burns. This is the primary use of the herb at this time. Some people smear the juice on cuts, scratches and bites.

Aloe vera was used as a purgative as early as the fourth century, B.C. This in no way makes it a "holy" plant. The liquid from the leaves was dried by the users and used as a purgative.

Aloe vera contains: barbaloin and isobarbaloin, forming "crystalline" aloin, 'amorphous' aloin, aloe-emodin, resin and volatile oil.

CAUTION: Excessive use of aloe vera as a purgative may cause hemorrhoids. Aloe should not be used during pregnancy.

This is called a Biblical herb and you should use caution when discussing this herb around the rural folks, and/or a man of the cloth. They may get nasty, as some of them believe that anything used in the Bible can do no harm.

AMERICAN CENTAURY (Sabatia angularis)

The American centaury (Rose pink/Bitterbloom) was used in the form of an infusion and tincture. The tincture was made by adding a handful of leaves and flowers to a quart of brandy and let it set for about two weeks. A tablespoonful of the tincture was given before each meal to improve appetite. Children were given a tablespoonful of the tincture each morning to rid them of worms.

An infusion was made to treat female complaints. Details were limited on this use.

ASPARAGUS (Asparagus officinalls)

Asparagus is a very well known garden vegetable. The roots, shoots and seeds were used in herbal medicine, and sometimes a syrup was made from the young shoots.

Asparagus was used as a: diuretic; diaphoretic; laxative, due to the high fibre content. It was also used for the treatment of dropsy, gout and rheumatism

To make an infusion from asparagus, place the roots in hot, but not boiling water for about two hours, then strain. Drink freely of this infusion for aid in dropsy and kidney affections, like stone or gravel in the kidneys or bladder. People made a syrup from the young shoots and gave four to six tablespoonfuls for a dose.

The young shoots eaten as a food have a powerful effect on the kidneys and is believed to have a sedative influence over the heart.

Advocates of herbal medicines would feed large amounts of asparagus shoots to the "old ones" in the belief that it would prevent them from going "silly."

Asparagus contains: Vitamins A, B1, and G; and the minerals calcium, iron, phosphorous, magnesium and trace minerals. It also contains a food fact called "asparagin," which was believed at one time to stop aging.

BINDWEED (Ipomoea pandurata)

The bindweed (Manroot/Wild potato) was more of an Indian herb. The early settlers learned of its medicinal use from the Indians. The dosage of the powdered root of the bindweed was two pinches as required. A decoction was made from the root to treat liver complaints, dyspepsia, gravel, dropsy and costiveness. A syrup was made from the bindweed root and mixed with other herbs to treat whooping cough, asthma and consumptive coughs. Little more could be learned about the use of this herb. It is no longer used in herbal medicine.

BAYBERRY (Myrica cerifera)

The most common local name for the bayberry is "waxberry." Nearly everyone has heard that the bayberry was used to make candles and soap. The wax is an edible fat.

The bayberry contains: (berries) myrica wax, comprising glycerides of palmitic, stearic and myristic acids, lauric acid, unsaturated fatty acids; (root bark) volatile oil, tannic acid, gallic acid, an acrid resin, myricine acid, an astringent resin, gum and starch. Action largely due to the resin content.

Uses of bayberry: astringent, weak diaphoretic, tonic and sialogoque.

An infusion was made from the bark for drinking or for use in poultices. Some old timers preferred making a decoction from the bark.

Herbal users believed the bayberry would remove "canker" from the system in all chronic cases. They also used the bayberry to make poultices to treat old sores, scrofulous tumors (T.B. or the glands), etc.

Some people drink an even mixture of bayberry and sumac bark make by decoction to treat scrofula in any stage.

One old lady said her family used the powdered bark of the bayberry as a snuff to treat "nose catarrh." She also said they chewed the bark to produce "spit", heal "bad gums" and help toothaches.

Herbal advocates used the bayberry as a gargle, douche, and as a poultice in the treatment of sore throats, leucorrhea and ulcers. They also used the bayberry internally to treat mucous colitis, diarrhea and feverish conditions.

Large doses emetic and may cause flatulence.

BAY TREE (Persea borbonia)

The sweet bay was used in herbal medicine by many people years back. The medicinal use of the sweet bay in now limited to a few of the older people. They know where the few remaining bay trees are located. The bay tree leaves were used for such things as cooking, confections, and liqueurs are now imported from some other region.

The sweet bay leaves contains: Volatile oil (1-3%) comprising geraniol, cineole, eugenol, terpenes; tannic acid and bitter principles. The berries contain fat (25%) and cineole.

The berries and leaves of the sweet bay were used as an antiseptic, stimulant, stomachic, weak insecticide and at on time used to stimulate digestion.

The sweet bay was used in some homes to make liniments. Many of the old-timers swear it will relieve rheumatic pains and sore joints.

Many of the rural folks put the dried leaves in and under the house to kill ticks and fleas. None of them ever said whether it worked or not.

In some areas the people made a weak tea from the sweet bay and used it as a social drinking not unlike sassafras tea. A much stronger tea of sweet bay was used to reduce fever and other like ailments.

The bay tree leaves are gathered in the early fall and hung up in bunches to dry in a shade. The tea was made from the dry bay leave.

BEECH (Fagus grandifolia)

Make a decoction of the bark of the beech for people with diabetes and to give children to control bed wetting. One cup of the decoction would be a dose.

A decoction made from the leaves of the beech is used for obstinate ulcers, skin diseases, headaches and low spirits.

BEECH DROPS (Epifagus virginiana)

This plant is a parasite that grows on the roots of the beech tree. It has a yellowish white to brown color, and just plain looks sickly. The root has a yellow color. It is about a foot tall, many has scales instead of leaves. Many flowers grow on the branches. This is an astringent and is used on ulcerous skin conditions.

The roots and tops are powdered and sprinkled on the place to be treated. A tea may be made and used as a wash. A combination of beech drops and cherry bark can be used to treat hemorrhages of the bowels. This combination also makes an excellent gargle for ulcers of the mouth.

Beech drops are known as cancer root by some folks. You will find that the beech drops parasites are very difficult to find.

CARAWAY (Carum Carui)

Caraway was cultivated in gardens. The seeds were used to treat people afflicted with flatulency or colic. A dose of the seed was one teaspoon level. The infusion is made of two teaspoons of caraway seeds to a pint of boiling water. Drink a cup of the infusion. I do not know of anyone who was able to make oil of caraway seeds. The real reason is they didn't have any use for the oil.

The herbs in this book is a history of their use only. Talk with a herbal expert before using any herb. Herbs contain real drugs, so you better use caution when dealing with them.

BITTERWEED (Helenium amarum)

The bitterweed is a pest plant despised by dairy farmers. When a cow eats the bitterweed, the milk given is also bitter. Many backwoods folks liked the bitterweed milk and claimed it would keep the milk from "blue johning." Blue johning is a stage milk goes through before clabbering when man or beast are inclined to pass it by.

Some of the old folks made a tea from the bitterweed and drank it as a liver tonic.

Colored people drank the bitterweed tea as a treatment for "sugar." (diabetes) A few other herbal users said they sometimes used the tea for that purpose.

Very little information was found on any other use of the bitterweed. A very limited number of herbal users treated fevers and measles with a tea made from the bitterweed.

BONESET (Eupatorium perfoliatum)

The boneset herbal plant (Thoroughwort/Fever/Indian sage) was at one time quite common in rural areas for the treatment of coughs and colds. A tea was made by infusion from the dried boneset plant. The dosage was one cup of the tea as needed. This plant has a very bitter taste. A tonic was made by decoction and used to treat other complaints.

The rural herbal users gave the tonic to "make them puke" (vomit) when someone had ate bad food or poison. (A large amount of the tonic)

Herbalists gave the tea for the "flu" and sometimes in the treatment of rheumatism or dropsy. The boneset was also used to reduce fever.

As with other herbs, the name indicate what a herb was used to treat. It must of been used in some way for broken bones

The boneset plant contains volatile oils; gum; resin;

gallic acid; tannin and a glucoside and eupatorine.

BLACKBERRY (Rubus louisianus)

The blackberry was the wonder herb of the backwoods. It was used in more ways than any other herb. The blackberry may be given in powder, infusion, decoction, syrup, extract and vinegar.

The blackberry (root, dried or fresh leaves and fruit) was given for the treatment of chronic diarrhea, dysentery, cholera infantum, summer complaint and cholera morbus.

The above complaints were treated by making a syrup from the bark of the blackberry root. Many others made a decoction by taking a half cup of the mashed root to a pint of water. The dosage of the decoction was three tablespoons four times a day.

The blackberry was also used as an astringent, tonic and diuretic.

Blackberry powder, most often used, was made by drying the fresh ripe berries in the sun or in the oven with low heat.

The berries were then ground to a powder with a "meat grinder" and placed in a jar with a tight lid. This was by far the best method of keeping the blackberries and having them ready to give as a medication any time of the year.

Herbal advocates gave the powder in the treatment of diarrhea, which was often referred to as "relaxed bowels" and the "runs."

The old timers made a tea by pouring about a pint of boiling water over a handful of blackberry leaves and steeped them for about four or five minutes. The dosage of this tea was a cup taken several times a day or until the case of the "runs" was stopped.

One can stop diarrhea by eating the fresh blackberries when they are in season.

Herbal practitioners soaked blackberry leaves in any hot wine to make an infusion. They then placed the hot leaves on ulcers twice a day until the ulcers were healed.

Herbal healers added blackberry jelly to hot water and used it as a gargle for sore throat. They would also use some of the other blackberry preparations when jelly was not available.

Some of the old timers would treat swelling of the limbs or dropsy by adding blackberry jelly to apple cider vinegar and using it as a compress

All the backwoods folks, would can many quarts of blackberries and blackberry juice to use in treatments for sick stomach or any other complaint causing distress at either end. Blackberries were used to stop vomiting.

Blackberries (fruit) contains vitamin C, organic acids, sugars and pectins: (leaves) contain tannins and other minerals.

RASPBERRY (Rubis Idaeus)

The raspberry is more of a female herb than any other use. An infusion is made from the leaves and given in small dosages during confinement to ease and speed parturition. Large dosage of leave infusion is given to ease painful menstruation. The leaf is also used to treat diarrhea. Large amount of the fruit is a mild laxative.

Raspberry leaf tea was given to reduce bleeding during childbirth. It was used for morning sickness.

Raspberry were crushed in apple cider vinegar and given diluted in water to treat or reduce fever or ease a sore throat.

Raspberry (leaf) contains fragarine and other substances, acting in isolation as both uterine muscle stimulants and relaxants. The fruit contains citric acid, vitamin C and pectin.

Raspberry (fresh or dried leaves, fruit) was used as an: astringent, oxytocic, nutritive and laxative.

BLACK HAW (Vibumum rufidulum)

Very knowledgeable herbalist used the black haw as an uterine tonic and sedative.

Black haw (root bark) is used as a: sedative, spasmodic and tonic tea.

Midwives made an extract from the root bark of the black haw. This extract had a very unpleasant taste, so it was "doctored" up with cinnamon water or some other good tasting herb.

Midwives believed the black haw extract would prevent miscarriage. They would give the extract thirty days before the date that the last miscarriage occurred in the previous pregnancy. The dosage given was about a teaspoon each day.

Some herbal users say one can get relief from aches and pains by eating the ripe (black) black haw berries. Be sure and spit the pits out.

The Black haw root extract was taken by females for most every type of female complaint (Female complaint meant just about everything dealing with the female reproductive cycle.)

The black haw (root bark) contains: tannins, isovalerianic acid, resin and viburnine.

CAUTION: Many people ate the ripe black haw berries as food while in the woods without the slightest ill effect. Be sure you know it is the Southern black haw. Some people claim the black haw berries are poisonous, but I think that is before they turn black. If you are not sure, leave them be.

CARROT (Daucus Carota)

Carrots were grown in garden, as wild carrots were difficult to obtain. Only the root was used from the garden grown.

Carrots in one form or another were used to treat many complaints, like eye problems, skin problems, glandular disturbances, infant diarrhea and to regulate the menstrual period. It was also used for hiccoughs, chronic coughs, kidney stones, cancerous ulcers and fissures of the nipples.

Poultices were made from either raw, grated carrots or cooked, mashed carrots for use on abscesses, cuts, wounds and inflammations.

Make a strong decoction and use to treat grave complaints and to help pass stones from the kidneys and bladder, It can be used on cancerous ulcers and fissures of the nipples.

The seed from wild carrots are useful to treat obstructed menses, hiccoughs, chronic coughs and dysentery. Make a strong decoction or tea from the seed of wild carrots and drink warm.

Carrots were grated into very small pieces and dried and stored for use when they were not in season. The dried carrots were used in soups in winter. The Carrot soup was believed to coat the stomach and "guts" to help soothe them.

Carrots retard bacteria growth that cause diarrhea and tends to inhibit the urge to "puke." (vomit) Carrots give some relief for sinus complaints.

Carrots are now known to contain Vitamins A, B, C, E, and K, as well as phosphorus, potassium and calcium.

CASTOR BEAN (Ricinius communis)

Castor oil is made from the castor bean, Castor oil was one of the most common cathartic used in herbal medicine, as is mild and certain in its action. Castor oil was purchased from the "big store." The castor oil was too dangerous for them to make at home, although the castor bean was given to dogs to "worm them."

Caster oil was given as a treatment by all herbal users to relieve obstinate constipation, colic strangulated hernia and piles. They also gave a very small dose of castor oil before bedtime to treat difficult coughs.

Caster oil was used as an enema to remove hard "stools."

Castor oil was used in many external home remedies as an emollient and as a vehicle for many ointments. The oil was also used to treat the eyes.

The castor bean (seed) contains: Protein (to 25%); fixed oil (to 50%); comprising ricinoleic, oleic, linoleic, stearic and hydroxystearic acids. One of the protein substances in the whole seed is a toxic albuminold, ricin to which the poisoning is due.

WARNING: The whole castor bean seeds are poisonous. Do not use them internally. Large doses of castor oil can cause vomiting, colic and a severe case of the "runs."

CATNIP (Nepeta Cataria)

Catnip, also called catmint and catwort is a common plant and was grown in the home garden or yard. It was used both as a tea and poultice.

Catnip (dried flowering plant) was used as an: antidiuretic, antispasmodic, stomachic, carminative, and weak emmenagogue.

The old timers used catnip tea to treat hysterical and nervous afflictions. They also gave the tea to produce "sweat" and as an aid for colds.

Some herbal users claim that by placing a catnip compress on the forehead, it would relieve pressure from the eyes and dull a headache. They also used the catnip to relieve the pain of a bee sting.

Mothers gave their infants catnip to relieve flatulency and colicky pain.

Poultices were used on too many complaints to list. This is a try and see cure as it just will not work on some people.

Midwives gave catnip for irritability and delayed menstruation. They also applied catnip to abrasions, cuts and bruises.

Some people mixed catnip, ground cloves and sassafras bark as a treatment for aching teeth.

Herbal specialists treated chronic bronchitis by the patient smoking catnip. This treatment may cause hallucinogenic effects and should not be tried.

Catnip contains: volatile oil comprising thymol, carvacrol, nepetol, nepetalactone and nepetalic acid, also tannic acid.

Antispasmodic action may be due to the oil content.

WARNING: Catnip is a mild hallucinogen when smoked. Do not try it.

AGRIMONY (Agrimonia SP.)
(Cocklebur/stickwort)

The rural folks in some areas were using the cocklebur (Xanthium strumarium) that grows in cotton fields, believing that it is the same as agrimony, or is agrimony. This is one of the dangers in herbal medicine. Know your herbs or do not us them.

The herbalist made a strong decoction from the root and plant of the agrimony. Sometimes sugar or honey was added to taste.

The most common use of agrimony is in the treatment of coughs and "belly complaints." In some areas, it was used to clean wounds.

A few of the older folks used the decoction for diarrhea and dysentery.

One herbal user said he added sugar and alum to agrimony and used it as a remedy for tapeworms.

The rural folks also used the agrimony decoction to treat scrofula, gravel, diabetes, and cystitis. Even sore throat and chronic catarrh were on their list.

Agrimony contains volatile oil, tannin, and resin. The combination is an antibiotic, astringent, and anti-inflammatory.

All the people on one rural road said they traded

"taters" to the root peddler for agrimony and other herbs. This may account for the fact that a given herb will be used all down one road and not on the next road.

CAYENNE PEPPER OR CAPSIUM
(Capsicum annum)

Cayenne pepper is grown in all section of Louisiana, and in sections of other states. You will have no problem locating it. "Capsicum" is the Greek work "to bite," and after you have tasted it, you will know just how well it will really bite. Cayenne is pungent and biting to the tongue although it is gentle in the stomach and is considered an internal stimulant.

Cayenne pepper is an irritant and local stimulant. When ingested in moderate doses, it gives a feeling of warmth, increases the secretions of the stomach and thus aids in digestion. It is given to drunkards to retard vomiting. Continuous local application can cause blistering. A tincture of cayenne pepper is frequently used in liniments to treat rheumatism, neuralgia, headaches, colic and many other complaints. The powder of cayenne is used to sprinkle over plasters to be used externally.

Cayenne is non-poisonous, and there is not reaction to it. It is a natural stimulant worthwhile for use on diarrhea or dysentery with bloody mucus and bad breath.

You may add a pinch to cooked or raw foods and a little more to hot soups or teas as an aid to digestion. Juices with a little cayenne added will increase alertness.

A gargle for sore throat is made by adding cayenne, cinnamon and salt to a low proof spirit. There is also an anti-flu mixture consisting of cayenne, salt and apple cider vinegar. Cayenne powder dusted on a wound will stop bleeding.

Some people claim cayenne mixed with water will stop internal bleeding; this I don't know about.

A few grains of cayenne placed on the gums and in a cavity will bite, but will temporary stop the pain.

Sprinkle powdered cayenne pepper in your shoes as it tends to keep the feet warm. You will also have red feet and the insides of your shoes will be red when you remove your shoes.

Cayenne may be taken by rolling the pepper inside of bread to make a pill. Should you try to take it raw, you will soon understand why you need to make a pill.

Now you can understand why so much cayenne pepper was strung and hung in kitchens.

Cayenne pepper contains: Capsaicin; capsaicin; alkaloids; Vitamin C, and palmitic acid. This is from an old chemical breakdown and may not be correct. Keep cayenne pepper out of the reach of babies and young children.

Be sure you have cayenne pepper. All red pepper is not cayenne and may do more harm than good.

CHICKWEED (Stellaria media)

The chickweed is a pest in the garden, Very few people would consider it a herbal plant. It is a prime source of food for birds and animals in the winter. Some of the country folks had to cook the eat this weed for food in very hard time.

The crushed chickweed was made into a poultice. The poultice was used to treat arthritic joints and rheumatism. This poultice was also used to relieve bruises.

The chickweed contains mineral salts including calcium and potassium salts; also saponins.

CHICORY (cichorlum Intybus)

Chicory has been used in Louisiana for centuries as a "coffee" and also as a coffee extender. The leaves were gathered very young and used as a vegetable by the rural folks who liked its strong taste.

Chicory (fresh leaf, root) was used as a: diuretic, weak tonic and laxative. Chicory has little medical use.

The old folks used chicory as an enema to detoxify the body when a strong and immediate result as needed.

A very old lady is to pick the flowers of the chicory plant early in the morning, place them in water and let them soaking the sun for some time. She strained and stored the water to treat people on a "crying spell," over possessive or just down right out critical of others. She said to just add the chicory flower water to the tea or coffee of the one you wish to treat.

Chicory contains: inulin, sugar, mineral salts, lipids, Vitamins B, C, K and P, bitter principles (sesquiterpenoid lactones) chiefly lactucine and lactupicrine.

Some folks say that chicory will protect the liver from the effects of excessive coffee drinking.

CAUTION: Excessive and continued use of chicory may impair the function of the retina. The blue chicory flowers will turn a yellow-white soon after the sun strikes them and close up.

RED CLOVER (Trifolium pratinse)

The Indians were the first to make use of red clover. They used it for food and in ointments of external sores and would drink red clover tea for skin diseases.

Red clover (dried flower-heads, fresh plant) was used for alterative, anti-spasmodic, expectorant and vulnerary.

The old folks boiled the red clover flowers in water for about ten minutes. They then strained the water from the flowers and continued to boil the water down to a syrup. This syrup was used to make plasters to treat old sores, ulcers, burns and skin complaints.

Some herbal users made an infusion of the red clover roots and give the infusion to correct "acid stomach" and to "clean the blood." They also used this infusion to wash "foul" sores and ulcers.

Other herbal users drank the red clover infusion to treat psoriasis and eczema.

Red Clover (flowers) contains: salicylic acid, coumaric acid, isorhamnetin, a phytosterol glucoside, trifolianol, a quercetin glucoside essential oil, a phenolic trifolianol an hydroxymethyloxyflavone, pratol, sugars, including phamnose, a plant oestrogen and coumestrol.

WARNING: Talk to your doctor before using any type of clover. Clover may delay blood coagulation. Farmers make sure their breed cows doesn't get anywhere near green clover. A rat poison is made from clover.

WHITE SWEET CLOVER (Melilotus alba) (White Melilot)

White clover is used as a fodder for farm animals. A

field of white clover is a great source for bees to increase the amount and quality of their honey.

White clover (cured fresh plant) is used as: nutritive, aromatic, stimulant and vulnerary.

Herbal people did not use white sweet clover very often; however, they did use white clover in ointments to treat skin complaints. White clover contains weak antibacterial power.

Very knowledgeable herbalists used white clover homeopathically.

White clover contains: coumarin and related substances, occasionally dicumarol (melitoxin) and fixed oil.

WARNING: White clover contains dicumarols which act as a vitamin K antagonist, thus reducing prothrombin synthesis which delays blood coagulation. It is used in rat poisons.

CORN SILK: Stigmata maidis, Zea Mays

Corn silk was used more than one might think. It was used in the form of a strong tea. It as used for irritable conditions of the urinary organs. Corn silk was used with agrimony to control bed wetting, and for treatment of kidney, bladder, and prostrate. Some folks smoked dried corn silk in their pipe. Could not find out why, maybe they didn't have any tobacco.

CUCUMBER TREE (Magnolis acuminata)

The cucumber tree does not share all the glory and use as other herbs in the South. The bark of the root and the fruit was used in herbal treatments. The powdered root bark dosage was about a teaspoonful. The tincture was most often used. It was make by placing the fruit in weak alcohol for a given time.

The herbal users have used the fruit or cucumber to treat dyspepsia and general debility for many years.

Herbalist used the bark and fruit prepared in the required form to give relief from pains of rheumatism.

Midwives gave a tonic of cucumber tree for treatment in obstinate cases of suppressed menstruation.

YELLOW SWEET CLOVER (Melilotus officinalls)
(Common Melilot)

Yellow clover is the most common of the clovers and is planted to feed or draw bees because it is very sweet.

Yellow sweet clover (dried flowering plant) is used for aromatic, carminative, expectorant, antithrombotic, antispasmodic and antibiotic.

Herbal specialists used a decoction of yellow sweet clover to "unstop blood veins." An antithrombotic preparation is now made commercially from yellow sweet corn, which should tend to prove that herbal users were on the right track.

Yellow sweet clover contains: coumarin, and related substances. Elements released on drying are: a glycoside, fixed oil and melilotic acid.

WARNING: Clover may delay blood coagulation.

CHERRY LAURAL (Prunus caroliniana)

The cherry laurel (Cherry bay) is common in the lower South and sometimes used as a hedge. It contains cyanide derivatives and is very poisonous.

The very old rural folks say the cherry laurel, at one time, was used in the treatment of vomiting and nausea. It was also used as an eye lotion. A very small quantity of cherry laurel as added to some poultices for relief of pain.

The cherry laurel contains the glycosides prulàurasin (laurocerasin) and prunase, which are decomposed in water by the enzyme prunase to release hydrogen cyanide, benz-aldehyde and glucose. **WARNING,** this plant is no longer used in herbal medicine as it is very poisonous.

COLLARD (Brassica, Cole Wort Family)

If any plant that saved people's lives was called a medical herb, then the collard would be the greatest medical herb of them all. The collard is normally grown through the summer and eaten in the fall and winter. During hard time, the rural folks survived on cornbread, collards and, if lucky hog jowl. Nearly every family of the backwoods had an ample supply of blackstrap "molasses" which is a rich source of calcium, phosphorus and iron, and they finished the meal by "sopping" some molasses. Would you believe this was a fairly healthy and body building diet?

The drawback to collards is double; it smells up the house while cooking, and literally fogs up the house after consumption, as it is a large gas producing food. (flatulence)

Nearly all the rural used the collard leaf to bring a boil to a head. They also used the collard leaf in the same manner to "draw" splinters, thorns, etc. to the surface so they could remove them. They folded the collard leaf and placed in over the area to be treated. It was tied and left in place until results were obtained.

Collard leaves were sometimes used as a poultice to treat sprains and aching joint.

Collard green soup was fed to babies with "bad" color.

DEER'S TONGUE (Trilisa odoratissima)

The deer's tongue (Vanilla-plant) was not used directly as a medicinal herb. The dried plant was used in sick rooms to hide odors. It was, at one time, used as a diuretic although they found that it was much too strong for this purpose. This plant contains coumarin which is responsible for the attractive scent.

COMFREY (Symphytum Officinale)
(Knitbone)

I was unable to locate comfrey growing in the wild in many areas. These areas must of obtained the herb from other places.

Comfrey was used as an: astringent, vulnerary, demulcent, cell-proliferant and sedative.

A decoction was prepared by using a handful of chopped comfrey roots to a quart of water. The herbal users gave about half a cup for a "round" of treatment for "belly" problems. This plant contains alkaloids, so I would recommend that comfrey not be used internally.

The comfrey plant is used externally as a lotion, poultice or decoction. The old folks and other herbal users claim that comfrey is outstanding for bruises, wounds, ulcerations, neuralgia, rheumatism and varicose veins.

A very old "granny" said she made a poultice of the

comfrey plant to place around broken bones to make them heal. The allantoin content probably helped the bones heal.

The comfrey plant contains: allantoin (to 0.8%), tannic acid, mucilage, resin, alkaloids: consollidine and symphytocynoglossine; sugars, essential oil and choline. **WARNING:** Do not use this plant internally. It contains alkaloids.

CORN

Corn was the dietary staple for all the rural farmers. Corn, along with beans/rice would be a healthy diet even today without the fats and etc. Corn meal was made into a soupy mush to feed ill folks. They also made a heavy mush of corn meal to use as poultices.

Sweet ears of corn was feed to people taking diuretics.

In hard time the people would pull the ears of young corn when it was not much more than the cob. They would chop it up and use it for food.

Corn contains protein, Vitamin B, iron and potassium along with some other minerals.

COTTON (Gossypium hirsutum)

Cotton, the white gold of the south at one time, was used in a limited way in herbal medicine.

Cotton (root bark, seed oil) was used as an: abortifacient and emmenagogue.

Midwives made a decoction from the root bark of the cotton plant. They used the cotton root bark decoction to treat metrorrhagia.

Some herbal users gave cotton seed oil as a lubricant "bowel cleaner." They also used the cotton seed oil for a base in external treatments.

Negro herbal users made a decoction of the bark of the cotton root and used it as an abortifacient during the slave period.

Cotton (root bark) contains: acid resin, dihydroxy benzoic acid, salicylic acid, fatty acids, ceryl alcohol, betaine, sugars, phytosterol and phenolic substances. **WARNING:** No part of the cotton plant should be used internally.

COLT'S FOOT (Tussilago farfara)

Colt's foot (Bll's foot/Flower velure) is a common weed in many sections of this country. Early settlers brought it into many areas where it took foot. A decoction was made from the dried leaves and flowers. A handful of the leaves were boiled in a quart of water until only a pint remained. This brew was strained and sweetened. The dosage was about a half of a cup.

The rural folks used the colt's food decoction in the treatment of coughs, bronchitis, and laryngitis.

Some of the older folks made a poultice to treat external sores and ulcers. Some of them mixed dry colt's foot leaves with their tobacco to prevent coughing.

DANDELION (Taraxacum officinate)

A full grown dandelion root is about a foot long and about the size of the little finger, and is full of milky, bitterish juice. The leaves of this plant is a favorite of many cultures for eating as a food. The leaves must be gathered young or they will be too bitter to eat.

The dandelion (fresh or dried roots, leaves and flowers) is used as a diuretic, cholagogue, choleretic laxative, bitter tonic and stomachic.

The dandelion is considered a cleansing tonic because the salts in the dandelion act to neutralize the acids in the blood.

Pick dandelion flowers and leaves late in the season when they are bitter to use in an infusion. An infusion is made by placing one handful of leaves and one handful of flowers to each quart of water and steep for about fifteen minutes. Add syrup or honey to your taste and strain the liquid off.

Herbal users gave the above infusion several times a day for the treatment of biliousness and to reduce swelling of the ankles.

The bitter dandelion root was used quite often in folk medicine and was used to stimulate a sluggish liver. Simmer a half cup of freshly sliced dandelion root to each quart of water until about half of the water is left. Strain and drink about one fourth cup for each treatment.

To make dandelion coffee, wash and dry some fresh dandelion roots. Grind the roots into a fine powder, and use about a spoon of the powder to a cup of hot water.

All of the herbal users used the dandelion coffee as a liver cleanser, and as a tonic for the pancreas, the spleen and the female organs. This is a very bitter drink you will suffer no side effect and no acid discomforts.

Some of the old folks said that dandelion root was used as part of a treatment for gallstones. I did not find any information on this treatment.

The leaves and tops of the dandelion are simmered in

a decoction and used as a poultice on breast abscesses. They were also used on boils and abscesses on other parts of the body.

The folks gave the dandelion tea (coffee) to promote appetite and improve digestion. They also gave it as a treatment for rheumatic complaints.

Dandelion contains: taraxacum, a bitter principle; taraxerin, an acrid resin; taraxerol; taraxasterol; 3:4 dioxylcinnamic acid; flavoxanthin; inulin; citrid acid; phenyloxy a cetic acid; riboflavin; sitosterol; sitosterin; stigmasterol; coumestrol; Vitamins B, C and provitamin A.

BLUE FLAG (iris vericolor)

Blue flag (Snake lily/Flag lily/Liver lily) root made by decoction was used to treat liver complaints, sore mouth, ulcers and dropsy. An infusion of the leaves were used to treat "kids" with worms and to "loosen their bowels." Some herbalist just made a syrup from the flowers to treat worms. The fresh dried root of the blue flag was ground into a powder and given in doses of pinches according to how much "loosening of the bowels" was required.

The fresh roots were beaten into a pulp and used as a poultice to treat felons and bruises.

Most of the folks said blue flag was "pioson" (poison) and a person would be "better off for health by not taken to it." Knowledgeable herbalist were about the only ones to use blue flag in herbal treatments.

DILL (Anethum graveolens)

Most of us today associate dill with dill pickles,

although dill is used in several herbal remedies. The seeds have a powerful, spicy odor and a moderately warm and pungent biting taste.

Uses of dill (dried ripe seed, fresh or dried leaf): carminative, stomachic, slightly stimulant.

Midwives made an infusion of the seed in boiling water and gave it to women immediately after confinement and also to increase milk flow in nursing mothers.

Herbal healers poured a cup of hot water over about a teaspoon of dill seed. They strained the seed from the tea and gave the tea to infants to reduce "colic" and "wind." They also placed the seed strained from the tea in bread and gave it to adults to aid "hardened bowel" stools.

Dill contains: oil of dill comprising, d-carvone; d-limonene;l some phellandrine.

DEVIL'S BIT (For information only)

Devil's bit is also called unicorn plant, blazing star, starwort, etc. None of the herbal users could locate one of these plants growing. The rural folks must of obtained the devil's bit from the "root man." They also claimed they learned of it healing powers from the Indians. The root was ground into a powder and the dosage was four pinches. A very old man said the Indians just chewed the root and swallowed the juice.

The folks gave the devil's bit to aid stomach complaints such as nausea and vomiting. They made a weak solution from the powder to relieve coughing.

Midwives claim it would prevent miscarriages in some women.

Some folks claimed the devil's bit would improve sex

drive.

DOGWOOD OR BOXWOOD (Cornus florida)

The bark of the root, stems and smaller branches of the dogwood was used as a good remedy for "bilious" disorders, jaundice, and "low spirits." The dry bark was used in this remedy as fresh bark is "rough" on the stomach. The infusion was the preferred method of using the dogwood.

A handful of the chopped bark was added to a pint of boiling water for the standard infusion. The dosage was to drink quantities according to its effect.

The ripe berries of the dogwood was infused in "spirits" to make a tonic bitters.

A toothbrush or snuff brush was made from the small stems of the dogwood. The stem is peeled and one end is chewed soft to make the brush.

ESSENTIAL OILS

An essential oil is the fragrant essence extracted from a fruit, flower or spice. All expensive perfumes are made from essential oils. A drop of flower oil can be used to perfume your body.

You can use the oils to add lasting aroma to sachets and potpourris. Some people add a few droops of essential oil to their bath to obtain a fragrant smell.

Some of the oils would be suitable for scenting candles. "Punks" soaked in citronella oil, dried and burnt will keep away bugs.

Essential oils should be used with care, as they are

very highly concentrated. Always test a small amount on your skin to determine if you are sensitive to that oil.

You should purchase your essential oil from a dealer as making your own oil is not very effective.

ELDER (Sambucus canadenis)

Elderberry wine is the first response you receive when the elder bush is discussed. It has many other uses. The dwarf elder (sambucus ebulus) is poisonous so you better be sure you have the correct elder.

The elder contains: essential oil: comprising terpenes; the glucosides, rutin and quercitrin; alkaloids; tannins; Vitamin C; mucilage; anthocyanins, and the combined action is diaphoretic.

Uses of the elder (fresh or dried flowers, fruit, leaves, root bark and stem pith): Diaphoretic; laxative, antispasmodic; diuretic; and emollient. Also, used to make a home dye.

The elder was used in combination with peppermint and yarrow for the treatment of colds and nasal catarrh in the form of a tea. The elder was used alone as a gargle for sore throat.

The elder combined with other remedies was believed to be of value for constipation, hemorrhoids, rheumatism, bronchitis and cystitis.

Elderberry jelly was used to cure constipation in children. The root is a very strong purgative and is very wise to leave the root to the experts. CAUTION: If you do not know how to use the Elderberry, leave it be.

ELDERBERRY FACE CLEANER

Take a cup of buttermilk and add four tablespoons of elder flowers to it. Bring to a light boil for about twenty minutes. Remove from heat and let soak for about two hours. Strain and use a cloth to clean the face with the liquid by light rubbing. The cleaner is gentle to the skin and very effective.

FENNEL (Anthemis cotula)

This herb was raised in the country garden as it was difficult to fine a source of fennel.

Uses of fennel (fresh and dried leaf, oil dried ripe fruit, rarely roots): Carminative; aromatic; weak diuretic; mild stimulant. Fennel seed was given for dyspepsia, difficult digestion, flatulency and colic in children.

WARNING: Large doses will disturb the nervous system.

Mash a teaspoon of fennel seeds and then pour about two cups of hot water over the seed. This tea was given by advocates of herbal use for regulation difficult and irregular menstrual periods. They would give this tea up to three times a day before and during the period.

The old folks believed that by eating fennel seed, it would increase milk while nursing.

Fennel seeds were used in conjunction with caraway seed and juniper berries to increase the flow of urine.

The fennel herb contains: Volatile oil, comprising mainly anethole and also fenchone, d-pinene, limonene, dipentene, phellandrene and anisic acid.

FOXGLOVE (Digitalis Purpurea)

Foxglove is given in this book for your information only as foxglove does not grow in many parts of the South. Pink foxglove grows wild in the Florida Parishes of Louisiana.

Purple foxglove is used as a cardiac tonic. The old folks used it for "dropsy" and pleurisy."

Foxglove contains: Several glycosides including digitoxin, digoxin and gitaloxin. Foxglove was, at one time, used as a poultice on wounds.

Purple foxglove makes a beautiful yard or pot flower, although it takes two years to bloom. WARNING: Do not attempt to use foxglove. (Digitalis Purpurea)

FRINGE TREE (Chionanthus virgincus)

(Snowdrop tree/Old man's Beard)

The fringe tree is a wild tree cultivated as an ornamental tree. It is recognized by its long white beard in the spring.

The fringe tree contains saponins; phyllyrin; and a lignan glycoside.

The fringe tree (dried root bark, fresh trunk bark) was used as a diuretic, hepatic, stimulant and cholagogue.

An infusion was made from the fringe tree bark. It was used as a tonic to treat any debilitating disease of hepatic origin.

This herb had limited use in folk medicine.

A poultice was made from the bark of the fringe tree and used to treat skin inflammations, ulcers, cuts and bruises. Very little reliable information could be obtained on the herbal use of the fringe tree.

FIG (Ficus carica)

The fig is mostly used as food and sometimes used in making home wine. In folk medicine it was used as a remedy for "stopped up bowels." It was also used as a poultice for boils and ulcers.

Some local people used figs to flavor or tone bitter coffee.

Another method required boiling four or five figs in a cup of water. Strain the liquid from the figs. Drink or gargle the fig liquid brew for a sore throat.

Green figs secrete a milky acrid liquid which is used in folk medicine to supposedly destroy warts.

To aid healing of gum boils, a fig was split and heated. Then, it was placed over the gum boil. This procedure was also effective for treating skin boils.

One old man said his family never ate figs as the seeds would stop up the "little guts" and kill you. (appendicitis?)

The fig contains grape (invert) sugar, gum, and sucrose.

GRAVEL ROOT (Eupatorium fistulosum)

The gravel root (Joe-pye weed) is a tall weed with a mass of purplish-white flowers. At one time, it was used as a dye. It is similar to boneset in chemical constituents.

The herbalist used the gravel root (dried root-stock) to lower fevers. It was also used in the treatment of kidney and bladder stones.

Many of the old folks used the gravel root to treat gout

and rheumatism. They said gravel root tea was useful in treating flu.

The gravel root contains volatile oil; a flavonoid, euparin; resin; an oleoresin, eupurpurin that is produced when poured into cold water.

GARLIC (Allium Sativum)

There is not question about the fact that garlic is one of the wonder herbs with many healing factors.

Garlic is known by its strong disagreeable taste and odor. It is like the onion, but you won't have any problem telling which is garlic. Folklore medicine tells and brags of garlic's great healing power and will lead a person to believe that it you used garlic, you would never become ill. I do know if you chew it raw, you will be able to terminate unwanted guests in short order.

Garlic can be prepared for use in many ways. It can be made into a syrup to control asthma, into a garlic oil for internal or external use, into garlic soup for restorative use, made into vinegar tincture for anti-epidemic body wash, and into an anti-rheumatic or anti-infection cider garlic drink, and as a poultice

Garlic is used to aid hypertension, draws out pain, and builds resistance to colds. It is vermifuge (removes worms from the system) and it tranquilizes.; Garlic is used with plenty of water as an enema for amoebic dysentery and can help treat mild cases of mononucleosis. (kissing disease)

Garlic is believed to be more effective on some types of bacteria than penicillin. Garlic soup will produce sleep in children.

To make a garlic soup, mash and simmer half a cup of

peeled garlic buds and add this to a good chicken soup. Cook the garlic and chicken soup about ten minutes and strain out the garlic buds. Serve the soup hot to prevent or relieve colds and other congestions. Chicken soup is known and proven to be a very good treatment for the common cold.

The British purchased garlic by the ton in World War I, as garlic is a strong antibiotic. They soaked spaghnum moss in diluted garlic juice and placed in on wounds to prevent sepsis. The Russians used garlic juice for the same purpose in World War II and they also used it as an anti-flu remedy.

To relieve pain from joints and toothaches, advocates of herbal medicine would use crushed garlic on gauze and apply to the area of pain. Some people took a sliver of garlic and placed it in the ear to stop earaches. I do not think this is a good method and should not be tried. Garlic is used to make poultices for boils and abscesses, and they would have to leave the poultice on for at least two day as garlic works much slower than drugs.

Garlic vinegar was used to clean a sickroom and you had better believe there would be a strong odor.

Herbal users would put garlic in most all the foods as they believe it would clean the entire system internally, help make the blood healthy while eliminating any bad germs, toxins or worms.

Recent laboratory experiments indicate garlic had the unique power to lower blood pressure. Some people claim that garlic and caraway seed will give relief for adult colic.

There are some indications that garlic will aid diabetes.

Garlic was roasted and applied to external areas to

relieve pain.

A recent four-year study by the University of Wisconsin has determined that by adding garlic, ginseng root or barley flour to diets may help increase life spans. The study has concluded that the spices and flour inhibit cholesterol accumulation in animals and may do the same in humans.

Bear in mind that these study groups get tax payers money for these studies and you can rest assured they will find something to get more money.

GOLDEN ROD (Solidago odora)

The medicinal golden rod may be identified by the taste of the flowers and leaves, which is similar to the taste of anise or fennel. This cure is given in warm infusion (do not boil) to produce perspiration, retard nausea and colic pains.

The old timers claim that by steeping a tea from equal parts of fresh golden rod and juniper berries, one could retard an allergic response to golden rod by taking a teaspoon of the tea for a month before the season. I wonder where they got the fresh golden rod before the season!

Some folk medicine advocates say that one can also take this tea to relieve kidney and bladder inflammation. I say, see a doctor first! Golden rod tea is also used as an aid in sleeping.

The dried flowering golden rod is used as an anti-inflammation, expectorant, vulnerary, astringent and is a weak diuretic.

Golden rod is most often applied externally in poultices or ointments to assist tissue healing. As a tea, it is used for internal tissue healing.

Flowering golden rod is sometimes used to treat chronic skin problems that are not allergenic.

Golden rod is also as assisting agent with other herbs for treating asthma, arthritis and rheumatism. Golden rod is not effective for diarrhea and may reduce cholesterol levels, although this has not been proven.

Golden rod contains flavonoids; tannins; saponins and organic acids. (such as: citric, tartaric, and oxalic) It also contains some unknown substances not yet analyzed.

HORSERADISH (Cochlearia armoracia)

This plant is cultivated in the home gardens. Horseradish grows spontaneously in gardens which may indicate that in bygone time someone had grown them as a medical herb. Horseradish produces irritation and is sometimes used in place of mustard in a poultice Horseradish produces perspiration and is also used in treatment of dropsy, rheumatism, neuralgia and other complaints

A warm infusion of this plant is made by using one-fourth cup of the root to a quart of water. Drink sufficient amounts to produce perspiration.

Horseradish is a potent stimulant and is used to clear nasal passages, drop fluid level in the system, a digestive aid and is said to cleanse the system of infections. A strong solution is held near the eyes to clean foreign objects from the eyes as it will produce plenty of tears.

Horseradish was used as one of the herbs in a mouthwash. Toothbrushes were also made from horseradish.

Rheumatism was treated by swallowing very small pieces of un-chewed horseradish root for about a month. Some old timers claim good results by this remedy.

Horseradish contains a glycoside, sinigrin, which will decompose in the presence of water by the enzyme myrosin which will produce mustard oil. (allyl isotheocyanate) The fresh root also contains Vitamin C and some antibiotic substance.

HORSE MINT (Monarda punctata)

The horse mint (Origanum/Dotted monarda) had very little use in herbal medicine. A strong decoction was made from the horse mint. It was used to treat complaints of difficulty in evacuating urine. It was also used in the treatment of gravel

Other uses of the horse mint could not be determined.

INDIAN PIPE (Monotropa uniflora)

Indian pipe is also known as fit root, bird's nest, ice plant.

Very little use of the Indian pipe herb is known. Very knowledgeable herbalists mixed the juice from the Indian pipe plant with water to treat sore eyes.

This plant possesses nervine properties. The expert herbal user pulverized the root of the Indian pipe and gave teaspoonful dosage for epilepsy and convulsions in children. **WARNING:** This plant is very dangerous and should not be used in any way or form.

ICE VINE

The "ice vine" as used to reduce fevers and in the making of a poultice to treat infections. Very few of the old timers ever heard of the "ice vine." Its use must have been limited to a very small region, or it is known by some other name in other sections.

HOLLYHOCK (Althaea rosea)

The hollyhock is cultivated in most areas for ornamental use. It is just a yard flower and its medicinal properties are no longer considered. Folks made a tea from hollyhock. This tea was used to treat inflammation of mucous surfaces in the throat, stomach, bowels, and urinary passages. Sometimes it was used to treat leucorrhea, and as a mouthwash. This is not first hand information, it is "Grandma said."

IRONWOOD (Ostrya virginiana)

Folk medicine does not make much use of the ironwood as only the heart of the tree is used. This tree is very hard and the heart is very difficult to recover.

An infusion is made from the chips of the heart of the tree. It was used on intermittent fevers, neuralgic affections, dyspepsia and scrofula. The dose is one teaspoon three times a day before meals.

JERUSALEM OAK (Ostra virginiana)

Jerusalem oak grown all over the United States. It is used for many different herbal treatments. This depends on the area where the herb is used as to what it is suppose to treat. It has an odor not unlike wormseed, although it may smell better.

Herbalist made an infusion from the Jerusalem oak.

The strength of the infusion doesn't have any standard among the users. The dosage is two tablespoonfuls as they see fit.

They used the Jerusalem oak in the treatment of asthma, worms, coughs, suppressed menses and consumption.

Many of the rural folks claim Jerusalem oak will rid the chicken house of mites and the house of fleas.

JIMPSON WEED (Datura Stramonium)
(Thorn Apple/Stink weed)

The prime use of the jimson weed by herbal users was in the treatment of bronchial asthma. The dry leaves were smoked in a cigarette, although most women smoked the jimson weed in a pipe.

Jimson weed (dried leaves) was used as an anti-spasmodic, narcotic and anodyne.

They sometimes mixed jimson weed and mullein leaves in treating asthma.

Some folks used the jimson weed as a poultice to reduce local pain.

The old timers treated their "piles" by rubbing the parts with the green jimson leaves after each "hocky."

The jimson weed contains alkaloids, comprising mainly of hyoscyamine, hyoscine, atropine, whose action relieves spasms of the bronchioles during asthma attacks.

The old folks used to sit out on their porches in a rocking chair. The younger members would light pipes with dried jimson weed and mullein and give to the old folks. When the old folks got up and started dancing around the chairs, they took the pipes away, as they now knew they had

enough for a dose.
WARNING: Jimson weed is poisonous and hallucinogenic. The jimson weed is very dangerous, even when used by herbal experts. Leave this herb be.

JUNIPER (Juniperus SP.)

Juniper is considered by many herbal users as the most curative of the simple herbs. The berries are gentle stimulant and diuretic although it will make the urine have a smell of violets. Juniper berries will act to aid the kidneys. Juniper may be used with most other herbs, except when one is trying to lower a fever. An elderly man said that juniper berry tea would get rid of colic and "poots." (flatulence)

Make a standard tincture and apply to any external painful swelling for relief.

Make a poultice of mashed juniper berries for relief of neuralgic pains, rheumatic pains or swellings.

Make a strong tea of the needles, wood or bark. Take frequent baths in the tea for rheumatism.

Juniper is used as an antiseptic, diuretic, stimulant, carminative, rubefacient and as a urinary antiseptic. Juniper is also used externally to stop bleeding and to treat wounds.

Juniper berries were roasted and used as a coffee substitute at one time.

INDIAN TURNIP (Arisaema triphyllum)

The Indian turnip (Jack-in-the-pulpit/dragon root) was dried and ground into a powder. The dosage was two pinches mixed with honey. The powder was mixed with syrup for some ailments.

Very knowledgeable herbalists gave the powdered Indian turnip for the treatment of coughs, asthma and consumption or the lungs.

The rural folks said it was used to treat "wind and bowel pains."

Midwives gave the Indian turnip for the treatment of "thrush." They used the powder and syrup mixture of the Indian turnip for the treatment of other mouth and throat complaints of the same nature as "thrush."

The Indian turnip has big expectorant properties, therefore it may be of value in other ailments.

LAVENDER (Lavendula Spica)

Lavender is grown in the home garden and is used in many ways in herbal folk medicine. It is most often used as a sedative, antiseptic, stimulant, weak diuretic and anti-spasmodic. It is also used to hide the bad smell of some herbal medicine.

Lavender is used internally as a mild sedative and cough suppressant, also colic. (flatulence) Lavender is used externally for relief of rheumatic pains. Lavender oil vapor is inhaled to prevent fainting and vertigo.

Lavender is used as an antiseptic rub or lotion for cuts and chapped hands.

Lavender oil is used as an insect repellent but I do believe it attracts some of them. Mosquitoes and mites seem to dislike the smell of lavender as they leave an area where lavender water is sprinkled. Women of the folk medicine period would wet a small rag in lavender water and carry in on their person to ward off insects, but I strongly believe it was for some other purpose.

Some of the old folks clam that lavender oil will stop a headache, minor "all overs" (mental depression) and neuralgic toothache.

Lavender contains linalol, linalyl acetate, hydroxycoumarin, limonene, cineole, geraniol and herniarin eucalyptol.

LEMON (Citrus Limonum)

The lemon today is so common that one would never believe that it was used in many herbal treatments. The lemon is used in folk medicine for anti-scorbutic, tonic, refrigerant, stimulant, carminative and an aromatic. The fresh peel and oil of lemon was used in many ways. The lemon peel is still used as a bitter, astringent and skin tonic along with other normal uses.

Lemon juice is used cold as a drink and hot as a treatment for colds. Small doses of lemon juice stimulates the stomach and facilitates digestion. It was also used to treat scurvy. Many other cures ascribed to the lemon has since been proven to be without foundation.

Some advocates claim that the drinking of moderate amounts of weak, un-sweetened lemon juice would cleanse the body of boils and other various skin problems. Another cure called for heating a lemon and then slitting the fruit. Salt was then added into the slit. One could insert an aching finger into the slit and hold it there until the pain was gone.

The lemon is used as a styptic to stop the flow of blood. It was also used to reduce fever.

Some people used the lemon to detoxify rheumatic and arthritic patients. Lemon juice is said to be useful in controlling some bladder and kidney infections.

Lemons were hard to come by in the far back rural areas of the herbal folk medicine period. People would procure a years supply when they made their yearly trip to the "big store," which could be a two days trip. They would store them by filling a jar full of the lemons and covering the jar's contents with lemon juice and salt. To prepare for storage procedure, each lemon was washed, scrubbed and dried. The lemons were then quartered from the tip to within half an inch of the bottom. Salt was placed in the lemon and pushed back together. Next, a tablespoon of salt was placed in the bottom of the jar. The lemons were pushed down into the jar adding salt after each lemon until the jar was full. Lemon juice was then poured into the jar to assure that all the lemons were covered. The jar was then sealed. The container was turned every day for about a monthly in a dark storage. The lemons would keep well for about a year. Don't know how they used the lemons with all that salt in them.

Lemons contain citric acid, hesperidin, pectin, Vitamin A, B and C, citral, citronellor, d-limonene, phellandrene and sesquiterpene.

LICORICE PLANT (Glycyrrhiza glabra)

Licorice has been used medicinally for 3000 years.

At an earlier time, every store had a jar of licorice candy. They were little black twisted sticks about five inches long. In fact this was about the only candy to be had at that time.

The older folks claimed that licorice candy would help prevent cancer and/or cure it. They were vague on what they really believed. The licorice plant contains an extract called glycyrrhizin. I believe they would of had to use the plant, not the candy.

Licorice was also used to treat coughs and bronchitis gastric ulcers: also has a mineralocorticoid action in treatment of Addison's disease. Used as a lotion for use on inflamed eyelids.

Licorice contains calcium and potassium salts of glycyrrhizic acid; flavonoid glycosides, liquiritoside and isoliquiritoside; sucrose and dextrose, starch, protein, fat; resin; asparagin, volatile oil; saponins.

LILY-OF-THE-VALLEY (Convallaria majalla)

(May lily)

The lily-of-the-valley may be found in yards throughout many areas. They are planted mostly as a yard flower now.

This herb contains cardia-active glycosides (cardenolides) similar to foxglove glycoside, especially convallatoxine, also convalloside, convallotoxole, and convallotoxoside; a saponoside, convallamarine.

The dried flowers of the lily-of-the-valley are used as a diuretic, emetic and cardiac tonic. It regulates heart action and is considered safer than foxglove.

This plant is poison and you must not try to use it.

LETTUCE (Lactuca Sativa)

The first thing we think of when lettuce is mentioned is hamburgers and salads. It also has other values as herbal medicine.

In the early backwoods environments (pre-1940), mothers nursing their babies would eat lots of lettuce, unaware of its real cause and effect. But, they were aware that this would quiet a baby down after nursing. Lately, scientists have discovered that mother's milk has a very small amount of opium in it, but who is to decide how much would be required to quiet a baby? They have also discovered that lettuce has a small amount of opium in it.

The juice of lettuce was prepared and kept for several other uses. It was used also for chronic rheumatism, colic, checking diarrhea and in relieving coughs. Lettuce juice was used on people with nervous conditions. A cloth wet with lettuce juice and placed on the forehead is said to relieve headaches. This was possible effective due to the opiate properties present in lettuce juice.

LIZARD'S TAIL (Saururus cernuus)

The lizard's tail (swamp lily) was a herbal plant that was used only as a poultice. The root of the lizard's tail was made into a poultice and applied to any inflamed or swelled surface.

Midwives roasted lizard's tail (root) and used it to treat complaints from women of pains in the breast, sore nipples, etc. They also used the poultices to treat lumbago.

It could not be determined how widespread the use of the lizard's tail was because so few herbalist ever used this herb.

LOBELIA (Lobelia SP.)

Also called Emetic herb, Indian tobacco, Wild tobacco, Puke weed and Asthma.

Lobelia is poisonous in every sense of the word and one should not use this plant in any form unless he is an expert in the field.

Uses of the dried fruiting plant: anti-asthmatic, expectorant, emetic and siaphoretic.

The Indians were the first to use lobelia by smoking the plant to relieve asthma and other related conditions.

In herbal medicine, lobelia was used for croup, tetanus, whooping cough and pulmonary diseases. The leaves, seeds and capsules are given in the form of powder or tincture. A dose of the powder was administered at one to four pinches. The tincture was given at no more than ten to fifteen drops.

For croup, a teaspoon of the tincture was given along with warm drinks of some simple herb tea until the patient "pukes." (vomits)

The tincture was used externally to relieve pain and irritation caused by rheumatism, bruises, bites and certain other conditions.

The lobelia herb contains: alkaloids; comprising of lobeline, lobelidine, lobelanine, isolobelanine. It also contains lobelic acid, inflatin, resin, fat, fixed oil, and caoutchouc (India rubber).

This plant is **POISONOUS**...and may be fatal. Large doses cause purgation, vomiting, convulsions, meduilary and respiratory depression. Leave this herb alone.

MARIGOLD (Calendula Officinalis)

The marigold is well known as an ornamental grown in a pot or garden as an insect repellent. It has many remarkable healing powers. The marigold has a rather disagreeable odor which will be lost in drying. The taste is bitter, salty rough.

Marigold (entire flower-heads, individual florets, and rarely the entire flowering plant) was used as a cholagogue; styptic; anti-inflammatory; vulnerary; antiseptic; and other uses. It was used for inflamed lymphatic nodes, duodenal ulcers and some inflammatory skin lesions. Advocates of herbal medicine also used the marigold externally for treatment of leg ulcers and as a lotion for conjuctivitis. Yellow dye was obtained by boiling the flowers.

The flowers were made into an infusion and given daily for low forms of fever, scrofula, jaundice and suppressed menstruation. Some people used it also to treat scarlet fever, measles, and to bring out the rash.

Many ladies of the rural area used the marigold infusion for chapped hands and in their bath to reduce body scars and to soothe varicose veins. Eczema was quire a problem during this period. The ladies also used marigold lotion to aid painful lesions caused by dry eczema and about every other herb they thought would give them relief.

Marigold, prepared for use in all the different methods, was used on open wounds, parts that would not heal, ulcers and a hemostatic after tooth extraction.

Female herbal users used marigold in a form of a douche for leukorrhea and trichomonas vaginitis.

A tincture of marigold was used to reduce the swelling and pain of a bee or wasp sting. A few used the tincture for broken skin, wounds and bleeding.

Others say that by steeping marigold petals in vinegar for about ten minutes and applying to a knee, one could get relief from sprains.

Surgeons during the Civil War used the marigold to stop bleeding and infections. It was also used during World

War I to clean wounds and stop post infection.

Marigold was used to cause perspiration during epidemics of measles and smallpox. It was also used for headaches and toothaches.

Marigold contains Volatile oil; a yellow resin; calendulin; saponins; a bitter principle; all of which will aid bile secretion and promote wound healing.

MAYWEED (Anthemis cotula)

The mayweed (Dog's fennel/Wild camomile), is similar to chamomile. The mayweed may be substituted for chamomile, however, it is weaker and does not taste as pleasant. The mayweed must be given in a very weak infusion, otherwise it will produce vomiting.

The rural folks used the mayweed internally to treat colds, fevers, rheumatism, and asthma. An infusion or decoction was made from the flowering tips of the may weed for internal use.

Herbalist gave the tonic in complaints where copious perspiration would be required. Even a weak tonic may produce nausea of the stomach.

Some folks used the mayweed infusion externally in warm baths. These baths were used to treat rheumatism, swellings, pain, hysterical fits and contusions.

Herbal healers gave a strong mayweed (flowering tops) tonic to produce vomiting in complaints where poison was ingested.

AMERICAN MANDRAKE (Podophyllum peltatum)
(May-apple)

The Indians used mandrake as an emetic. The fruit of the mandrake was eaten, knowing that they would get the "runs" from eating the fruit.

Mandrake (may-apple) was used as a powerful purgative, gastro-intestinal irritant, antihelminic and antimitotic.

The mandrake root is dried and ground to a powder. The average dosage of the powder was about two pinches. Herbal users used the mandrake powder to treat chronic diseases, such as bilious and dyspeptic complaints. Venereal treatment was not effective.

The old timers used the mandrake to control the flow of urine.

Very knowledgeable herbalist added mandrake alcoholic tincture to water to produce podophyllin or podophyllum resin. This was used externally to treat soft venereal and other warts.

American mandrake (may-apple) contains podophyllotoxin, picropodophyllin, quercetin, pelatin, starch and flavonoids. WARNING: Mandrake is poisonous. External application must be carefully restricted to abnormal tissue only. Not to be used during pregnancy. You are well advised to leave this herb be.

BUTTON SNAKE ROOT (Eryngium yuccifolium michx.)
(Merrye Curvye/rattlesnake-master)

"Merry-e curvye" was the mysterious herb used in Louisiana herbal medicine. The correct name of the herb is now established. (Button snake root) "Merrye curvye" is colloquial, so bear this in mind when inquiring about this herb. The only information I found on the name was that a "Granny women" with the name of Mary Curby brought the plant to the attention of the local folks. Not knowing any other name, they called it merrye curvye plant. Everyone having knowledge of this herb made a tea from the roots. They used the tea to treat hives, whooping cough, measles and other throat complaints.

Some folks made a tincture from the merrye curvye. These people claimed that they painted the throat of their children to cure diphtheria. They claim this saved the lives of their children sometime around 1930. This treatment may have their children, but it sure was hard on cats as they believed that cats gave children diphtheria. They also believed that cats stole the breath of their babies, so what's new?

The "furrin" (from some other place) root man was paying very high prices for the "merrye curvye" roots. When considering that a days wages was fifty cents at that time, many of the farmers let their crops suffer to cash in on the "big money." NOTE: "Merrye curvye" is button snake root.

MILKWEED (Asclepias SP.)

Herbal users made a decoction of the milkweed by foiling a handful of the dried root in about three quarts of water. They gave about a half cup of the decoction, four times each day for the treatment of dropsy. They would give more or less according to the effect.

PLEURISY ROOT (Asclepias tuberosa)

Uses of butterfly milk weed (dried root stock): Diaphoretic; anti-spasmodic; carminative; expectorant. Also used in infections of the respiratory tract, such as Pleurisy. They used powdered root as a poultice on open sores.

Butterfly milk weed contains glycosides, including asclepiadin; resins; and volatile oil. **WARNING:** Large doses cause diarrhea and vomiting. Fresh leaf tea also causes vomiting.

MISTLETOE (Phoradendron tomentosum)

Mistletoe berries were used for people who had fits. (epilepsy) The berries were gathered around the end of November. They were dried and ground into fine powder, placed in a bottle with a good stopper so it would not be exposed to air. The dose was a thimble full four times a day. It was increased or decreased according to effects it had on the "victim." The powder was also given to dogs that had fits.

Mistletoe is very dangerous, so do not experiment with it in any way.

BELLWORT (Uvularia perfoliate)

The early settlers learned of the bellwort (Mohawk weed) from the Indians. The rural folks made a decoction from the root of the bellwort. The dosage was as required. The root of the bellwort was powdered and mixed with "hog lard" to be used as an external ointment or poultice.

The Indians used the bellwort for rattlesnake bites,

wounds and sores. Most Indians used the bellwort in raw form only.

The rural hunters chewed the root and swallowed the juice for sore throat. They said it was good for some bites and stings.

The rural folks used the bellwort for "bad gums & eyes." A few used bellwort in the treatment of erysipelas.

The herbal folks treated external "tainted" sores and wounds with both the bellwort ointment and poultice.

MULLEIN (Verbascum Thapsus)

Mullein is plentiful in all rural areas. Mullein was used in, or in combination with, many herbal remedies. This was probably because it was easy to obtain, and therefore, was tried more in herbal medicine.

Mullein (dried or fresh leaves, dried flowers) was used as an emollient; weakly sedative; expectorant; and the most common use was in the treatment of respiratory disorders. The flowers provided a pale yellow dye.

Quite a few of the folks would make an infusion of the leaves and flowers and use it to treat looseness of the bowels; diarrhea, colic; scalding urine and as an aid in the treatment of consumption.

Herbal users took the leaves and pith of the stalk and made a poultice. They would use the poultice on white swellings, sprains and inflammations.

Other people boiled the leaves of mullein in vinegar and applied the leaves to offensive sores, swellings and contracted sinews. The steamed leaves were used to treat hemorrhoids.

An eye wash was made by soaking mullein flowers in

rose water. It was used for a wash for that they called "weak eyes."

Many of the people would smoke the dried leaves alone or with other herbs or tobacco to help relieve long-time coughs and to help relieve nasal and chest irritations. It was smoked for asthma and worked well on many.

Some of the folks of that time would soak olive oil and mullein blooms and use it for earache and dry eczema. Some claim this same oil would control bed wetting in children.

A tea was made from the bloom just to drink.

Mullein contains mucilage; essential oil and saponites.

MUSTARD (Sinapis Alba)

Mustard with hot dogs is the most known use of this herb today. Many yesterdays' back, mustard was used to treat various complaints.

Mustard (leaves, seed) was used for a stimulant, irritant, emetic and preservative.

The most important source of iron for the herbal period was "mustard greens." Sometimes "cornbread" and mustard greens was their only available food. Mustard greens, when eaten, produced plenty of gas and foul odor. They also caused "loose bowels" and some un-scheduled trips to the outhouse.

Mustard seeds were used to make external plasters. A mustard plaster was used by herbal folks for just about every type of external. To make a mustard plaster, they would beat the white of an egg and add a little flour. They would then add ground mustard seed so as to make a soft paste. A cloth would then be placed between the body and the mustard paste, as mustard will blister.

They treated late stages of typhus fever, cholera and many other ailments by placing a mustard poultice on the belly. It was also placed on the chest for congestion.

They would used mustard foot baths to induce sweating and they also believed this would draw the blood away from the brain and other organs when in a congested state.

Ground mustard seed was used to preserve some types of food as it is a powerful preservative, prevents mold and bacterial growth.

Mustard contains a glycoside comprising sinalbin, an enzyme, myrosin, which interact in the presence of cold water when the seed is mashed.

STINGING NETTLE (SP.)

The nettle is a common plant and will give a painful sting when touched. This herbal plant was used to treat many complaints. Leaves were cooked as food in hard times.

The old timers had several methods to stop the sting of the nettle. One was to "piss" on the sting. Another method was to take the juice from the nettle and smear on the sting. They also claim yellow dock will stop the sting very fast. Today, one could use a weak ammonia water to kill the sting.

The nettle (fresh or dried leaves) was used as an astringent, anti-hemorrhagic, diuretic, galactagogue.

They ground the dry nettle leaves and used it like a snuff to stop nosebleeds. They used the juice to treat gravel complaints, internal hemorrhage and spitting of blood, a decoction to treat "bloody piss" and early consumption.

They would sweeten the decoction to treat diarrhea and dysentery.

The family was to use the nettle was to make a strong syrup using the nettle, wild cherry and blackberry root. They would boil the above in a quart of water for about twenty minutes and strain the liquid off. They would then add two cups of sugar and a cup of brandy or wine, stir well and place in a jar. The dosage of the syrup was a teaspoon full for very young children and a quarter of a cup for adults given about five times each day. They gave a laxative before giving the syrup.

Some people used the nettle to treat "sugar" and "high blood." Herbal quacks claimed nettles would grow hair.

The nettle (leaves) contains histamine, acetylcholine, formic aid, gallic acid, tannins, 5-hydroxtryptamine, Vitamin A and C, mineral salts, including calcium, potassium, silicon, iron, manganese and sulphur and other active substances and unknown components. There are many types of nettles, so you better be sure of the type you use.

NEW JERSEY TEA (Ceanothus americanus)

The root bark of the New Jersey tea has the smell and taste of peach leaves. It will turn water red. The stems, leaves and seed are made into a decoction or a strong infusion. The dosage is a cup three time a day. A Tincture is made from the bark of the root. The dosage of the tincture is a teaspoonful four time a day.

Herbalist gave a decoction of the New Jersey tea as a remedy for syphilitic complaints and gonorrheal discharges, although they indicated the results were poor.

They also gave the decoction to give relief from consumption and other diseases of the lungs.

A few rural folks claimed the infusion would control epilepsy, asthma and chronic bronchitis. They said it was also good for "dry coughs."

OKRA (Abilmoschus Esculentus)

Okra is mostly used as a food. Okra was boiled and fed to anyone with a sore or raw stomach. It was also used by anyone who had "low blood." According to some medical journals, the dried extract from okra can be used as a blood plasma by recombining with a liquid.

Herbal healers took the slimy extract from raw okra and used it to soften hard scabs and to soothe cuts, scratches and chapped hands.

The dried powdered okra pods was placed on cuts or wounds to retard or stop bleeding. They would bind a clothe over the powdered okra on heavy bleeding.

Okra is a very find food and should not be passed by.

OATS (Avena sativa)

Oats have long been used as a food for both man and animals. Oats (seed) were used in the treatment of debility because it was highly nutritious. The seeds were cooked into a thick mush and used as a poultice base for other herbs. A tea was made from the straw. The purpose of the tea could not be determined. Mush was also made from the oat seeds and mixed with other herbs to be used as a face treatment by the rural women.

Some folks said you must eat plenty of oats to keep

the bowels clean.

The oat seeds contain protein; gluten; starch; albumen, gum oil; salts and tocopherol.

ONION (Allium Cepa)

You are receiving medication each time onion is eaten raw or as a season in other foods. The onion is used for many other herbal treatments.

Uses of the (fresh bulb, fresh juice): Antibiotic, diuretic, expectorant, hypotensive, stomachic, anti-spasmodic, hypoglycaemic.

The onion was and still used by many people in the treatment of colds, bronchitis, coughs, laryngitis and gastroenteritis. A few folks used the onion because they believe it will reduce blood pressure and "sugar" level.

Many old timers roasted and split the onion and placed in on boils and tumors to bring it to a "head" and reduce the pain. They also mixed the onion juice in syrup, or made a syrup from onion juice and sugar. The onion syrup was given for colds and croup. These same old folks claimed the onion was good in "dropsies," suppression of urine, gravel, etc.

A common remedy to relieve "stopped up" nose or sinus was to inhale freshly cut onions.

Some users of herbs, mashed onions and placed them on protruding or inflamed hemorrhoids for relief of pain. They did not way whether it was an aid in healing.

Hunters of yesterday would mash onions and salt to apply to frostbite (chilblains) when the skin was not broken and mashed onions without salt should the skin be broken.

Mashed onions was applied to bruises to relieve pain.

Roasted onion poultices were applied to the chest to relieve cough or congestion.

The contents of the onion are similar to those of garlic, also containing glucokinins, pectin flavonoid, glycosides, Vitamins A, B1, B2, B5, C, E, Nicotinamide.

PEONY (Paeonia officinalis)

The peony was grown by the early settlers for medicinal use. The peony became a yard flower when its herbal use declined. It is not longer used in herbal medicine as the rural folks consider it to be poison.

The dried root of the peony was used as a sedative, diuretic and vasoconstrictor. It was used by midwives and very knowledgeable herbalists. Not many folks would even attempt to use the peony.

Midwives would use the peony to speed uterine contractions and slow down bleeding after childbirth.

Herbalist used the peony to treat kidney and bladder stones. They rarely used it in the treatment of varicose veins and hemorrhoids because of the side effects of the peony.

The peony contains and alkaloid; a detone, paconol, benzoic acid (5%); 1-asparagin; essential oil and a heteroside.
WARNING: Do not attempt to use the peony in herbal medicine.

PASSION FLOWER (Passiflora incarnata)

The passion flower is know as the maypop in many areas. Many a cotton picker had paused to fill their hungry bellies with the ripe maypop fruit growing wild in the cotton field. Some religious folks called the maypop flower a holy flower after the supposed symbolic association between the anatomical and numerical arrangement of the flower and the elements of the crucifixion.

The maypop (dried fruiting and flowering tops, fruit) was used as an anti-spasmodic, sedative and anodyne.

Very knowledgeable herbalists used the maypop infusion to treat nervous tachyacardia, anxiety and insomnia. They sometimes used the maypop to treat convulsions and epilepsy.

Most folks just used the maypop fruit as a tea tonic and sleep aid.

The maypop contains (fruit) ascorbic acid, flavonoids, citric and malic acids, amylopectin and fixed oil: (flowering plant) contains alkaloids comprising harmine, harmol, passitlorine, a cyanogenic heteroside, also flavonoids, passiflortannoid and maracutin. Eating the ripe fruit will do you no harm, but will make you sleepy. Note: Maypop contains a sedative.

PARTRIDGE BERRY (Mitchella repens)

The partridge berry (Tea berry/Squaw vine/Winter clover) was first used by Indians to lessen the pain of childbirth. An infusion (herb and berries) was used for the treatments by the rural people.

Herbalists gave the tea berry as an aid in treating dropsy, gout, and to increase urine flow. The infusion was also given two or three weeks before childbirth to reduce labor pains.

PEACH TREE (Prunus persic)

The dried peach stewed with sugar was used throughout the years as a laxative. The peach stew was given to the very old that was troubled with chronic "costiveness." (constipation)

Herbal specialists made a syrup of the peach seed kernels. They used this syrup to tone the stomach, bowels and the digestive system, They made a tincture of the kernels and used it to treat fever, debility and leucorrhea. The dosage of the peach kernel tincture was a teaspoon three time each day. WARNING: Do not use the peach kernel for any internal use. They are poisonous and dangerous.

The old folks made a tea from the peach kernels and used it for external use only. They used the tea for healing, cleaning and to retard the pain from wounds. The peach pits were cooked and placed in glycerine to preserve the tea for off season.

Some of the mothers poured a cup of boiling water over a cup of peach leaves and used the water to make a paste. This paste was applied to their children's "bellies" for about half an hour to get rid of the "worms."

PERSIMMON (Diospyros virginiana)

The persimmon is a very good source of food. The ripe persimmons were used to fill many a "belly during the hard time year." Some people made "spirits" from the ripe persimmons.

Most of the herbal users made an infusion of syrup from the green persimmons. The green persimmon infusion was used to treat diarrhea, chronic dysentery and hemorrhage of the womb. The dosage was given according to the size of the patient.

A decoction was made from the persimmon bark and used to gargle in ulcerated sore throat.

During the late 1920's, there was a severe outbreak of the "bloody flux" among infants, also known as "spotted spurge."

Nearly all the infants treated by a doctor died. The backwoods folks made a decoction of persimmon bark and added water to make a tea. They gave the tea to the infants day and night. None of their infants died. Some of them gave "first mother's milk" along with the tea and it seemed to speed up recovery. The persimmon bark tea work well on all ages to cure the "runs." It still will work.

PINK ROOT (Spigella marilandica)

The pink root was used by Indians as a herb to rid the tribe of round-worms. Herbalists picked up this remedy an improved the treatment by giving a purgative along with the pink root.

People , who used the pink root, gave a very small amount of the powdered root in the treatment of nervous headaches.

Some of the backwoods folks claim it is good for the treatment of the "all overs." They give just a pinch of the powdered pink root. Anytime any dosage is measured in pinches, you better take notice. The pink root is a narcotic and should be left to people who know how to use it.

POISON HEMLOCK

(Conium maculatum & Cicuta maculata)

The poison hemlock is a herbal plant that only herbal specialists should ever attempt to use in herbal medicine. This plant has the smell of mice urine. This smell should be enough to ward off the new herbalist. The dosage of the extract was one drop twice a day. A fomentation was made by adding a handful of leaves to a quart of boiling water. This was used on local external areas.

The older folks said poison hemlock was used as the last "cure."

The powdered hemlock was given to treat epilepsy, neuralgia, convulsions, hydrophobia and lockjaw.

Other old timers said a smidgen of poison hemlock would give relief for whooping cough, spasmodic laryngitis, and asthma. These old timers said they would never use poison hemlock to treat their own folks.

A few herbal users mixed a handful of hemlock with wax and caster oil. This was heated and spread on a piece of cowhide. The hide was placed on external tumors for treatment. Poison hemlock is no longer used in herbal medicine.

The poison hemlock contains several alkaloids, chiefly conline, which is the reason for the toxicity of all parts of this plant; paraconine; oil of conium; methylconline; conic acid and conydrine. NOTE: Any plant that contains an alkaloid must be handled with care.

The poison hemlock was used in the long past history of Athenian State as the poison for executions.

POKE WEED (Phytolacca americana)

(Coakum/Pigeon berry)

Nearly everyone has heard of "poke salad," but few have learned of the many herbal uses. Poke was first used by herbal advocates as an emetic and for treatment of venereal.

Uses of poke weed (dried root, young cooked leaves): emetic; purgative; narcotic; sternutatory; molluscicidal; spermicidal; fungicide; anti-rheumatic; and anti-catarrhal.

They powdered the dry poke root mixed with slippery elm to disperse scrofulous and hard abscesses. Some just roasted the root and applied it to the abscess. They also took the powdered poke root mixed with blood root and used the mixture to treat polyps of the nose.

They treated chronic and syphilitic rheumatism with the juice of the poke weed. One tablespoon was given every four hours. They made a strong decoction of equal parts from poke root, blood root, and sumac bark and used the decoction in the treatment of cancer and ulcers of the womb.

A few herbal users made an ointment of poultice to treat fungal infections, ulcers, hemorrhoids, and scabies.

Midwives applied the ripe berry juice externally to ulcers, tumors and sometimes used in childbirth. Many say this treatment is not very effective.

Poke weed mitogen factor (PWM) is employed for immunological purposes in modern medicine.

The poke root contains neutral principle, phytolaccin; alkaloidal substance; phytolaccine; phytolaccatonin (cyanchotoxin) and a hydrolysis product; phytolaccagenin; jaligonic acid; carboxyl and dicarboxy oleanenes; various steroids and saponins; potassium salts.

The poke berries contain saponins; mucilage; tannic acid; phytolaccinic acid; red pigment; caryophylline. The poke leaf contains antiviral protein called PAP and similar to interferon; rubber, fatty oil; and other chemicals not known at this time.

Some chemical elements of the poke weed is now being tried on Aids. (Interferon?)

The poke weed is toxic and dangerous!

The old folks made poke salad by soaking in salt water and cooked well with two changes of water. They used only the young tender leaves. They did not use and part of the stem of the poke weed. They never used any part with red on it.

The poke weed can cause hematological abnormalities, violent emesis and possible death.

PURSLANE (Portulaca oleracea)

This herb grows wild in yards and gardens. At a much earlier time, it was found only around ship ports, or at least, they never looked anywhere else.

The purslane has a very high content of Vitamin C. It was used aboard the ships to prevent scurvy.. In later years, rural herbal users grew purslane in their gardens. It was used for medicinal treatments and also was cooked with other vegetables as a food.

Purslane was used to treat scurvy, pulmonary and skin diseases.

Rural folks used purslane to "prod the heart for folks who was cold in summer." (Low blood pressure?)

Purslane contains Vitamin C, potassium salts, oxalic acid, urea, carotenoid pigments, alkaloids, glucoside, sitosterol, volatile oil, resins, organic acids, and sacchariferoid.

POMEGRANATE (Punica granatum)

Pomegranate is known to most people today as a funny looking fruit full of seed and sold in the supermarket every now and then. The pomegranate was imported to this country and grown as a herbal plant years ago. Some of the old bushes still grow in rural areas.

Herbal users took two small handfuls of bark of the pomegranate and chopped it into small bits. They would let it sit overnight in about two quarts of water. They would boil it down to about a pint and half and strain. The patient was given three doses about an hour apart, without the patient taking any food. This decoction was used to get rid of tapeworms. The patient was given a large dose of castor oil as soon as colic pains began.

Pomegranate (dried fruit rind, dried bark, fresh leaf, fresh fruit) was used for: astringent; antihelmintic; antibacterial.

Folk medicine people made a decoction of the pomegranate rind and used the decoction for the treatment of dysentery and diarrhea. They made an infusion of the rind for colic and stomachaches.

Herbal advocates made a tea from the rind and it was used as a douche in leucorrhea.

Some of the old folks steamed the leaves and applied them to external sores. The leaf has an antibacterial properties.

Pomegranate contains: (fruit rind) gallotannic acid; (root bark) alkaloids, comprising pelletierine; pseudopeiletierine; sopelletierine; and methylisopelletierine; (fruit) invert sugar, glucose; citric acid; boric acid; Vitamin C.

PRICKLY ASH (Zanthoyxylum clava-herculis)
(Toothache Tree)

The Indians and herbal users took the inter bark of the prickly ash and would pound it to a pulp. This pulp was placed on the spot of the toothache in order to kill the pain. This treatment would alleviate the pain, but did little to heal the disorder.

Prickly ash (dried stem and root bark, rarely fruit) was commonly used as: a stimulant, a diaphoretic and a carminative.

The boiled half-a-handful of dried bark in a quart of water until about a third of the water was rendered in preparing the decoction of prickly ash. They gave the patient about four tablespoons of the decoction every four hours for the treatment of chronic rheumatism.

Prickly ash contains: resins; alkaloid-like substance, a phenol, and xanthoxlin. NOTICE: It would be wise to leave the prickly ash remedies to the more experienced herbal users. However, if one must experiment, then take a small piece of the inter bark and touch it to your tongue. You will find it works and works fast.

PUMPKIN (Cucurbita pepo)

Most of the people know that the pumpkin is used to make pies. Others believe that the pumpkin is grown to have funny faces cut in them for Halloween.

Folks made a tea from the pumpkin seed to get rid of

the tape worm. They also gave the tea as a remedy for the "hot piss" complaint.

Many mothers gave pumpkin seed tea to their infants to keep them from wetting the bed at night. Some people parch pumpkin seed just to eat.

Other than food, there is little else known about the use of the pumpkin. When younger children would as their mother why some women had a large belly, she would tell them the woman ate a pumpkin seed. Needless to say, children shied away from the pumpkin seed. And, for the ones of you that never learned the truth, pumpkin seed does not make a woman's belly large.

POLYPODY ROOT (Polypodium polypodioides) (Brake Root)

This fern-type plant will be found mostly on decaying logs. This herb was seldom used in herbal medicine..

It was used as a laxative and expectorant. The common use was in treating chest complaints, coughs, and bronchial catarrh. It was also used as a tapeworm remedy, though not very effective.

Folks say a weak tea of brake root will "make them eat."

Polypody root contains essential oil; sugars; mucilage; bitter resins; tannic acid; a saponoside; polypodine; and mineral salts.

An infusion was made from the brake root by adding a tablespoon of the powdered root to a quart of boiling water. Sweeten to taste. The dosage was a pint in twenty-four hours.

RATTLE BOX (Daubentonia lexana Pierce)
(Coffebean)

A few of the rural folks used the seeds from the coffeebean in the treatment of tumors, growths, and sometimes "bad blood" in children. The extract was prepared by two-step process.

The coffeebean extract was prepared by crushing the seed and steeping in water for several hours. The water was drained from the seeds. The seeds were soaked in spirits for about a day. The seeds were strained from the spirits and discarded, leaving a strong extract. Several drops of the extract was given in a glass of water as a daily dosage.

The length of this treatment or the results of the treatment could not be accurately determined. Some claimed it cured their tumor, others claimed it only helped, and still some said it just didn't work for them.

The rattlebean seeds contain a chemical known as sesbanimide, similar to the antibiotic cychoheximide.

The farmers said the coffeebean was poison to livestock.

RUE (Ruta graveolens)

Very knowledgeable herbalist cultivated rue in their gardens. Rue is a very dangerous herb and the following data is given for your information only. You should not use or attempt to use rue in any way or form.

Rue was used as an: emmenagogue, abortifacient, antihelmintic, stomachic and diaphoretic.

Very knowledgeable herbalist gave a very small dosage of rue for relief of dysmenorrhoea, and also epilepsy.

They used rue externally to treat skin diseases, rheumatism, and as an eye wash. In some cases, rue was used as a gargle.

Rue was used on snakebites as it has the ability to expel poisons from the system.

Rue contains Volatile oil (.06%), and various ketones, including metnyinonylketone (to 90%). It also contains limonene, cineol methylacetate, resin, tannins, the rhamoglucoside, rutin, coumarin, fixed oil, bergapten, xantoxin, the alkaloids, ascorbic, furo-courmarins, and several other active substances. Warning: Rue is toxic. It produces mental confusion and can cause death. Pregnant women must not use or handle rue.

SAGE (Salvia SP.)

Sage is well-known in all parts of this country. Most of us think of it as a seasoning for meats. In folk medicine, it was used for many treatments or cures.

Sage (fresh, dried leaves or oil) is used as an antiseptic, antifungal, anti-inflammatory, astringent, carminative, emmenagogue, choleretic, ad weak hypoglycaemic.

Nearly everyone made an infusion of the sages leaves, called "sage tea." "Sage tea" was given for the treatment of summer complaints and worms in children. It was a popular remedy for coughs, colds, and sore throats for all ages. Sage tea was used as a gargle in treating "thrush or quinsy."

The most common use of sage was to use sage tea to induce sweating, although many users also claimed sage would reduce excessive sweating.

Midwives gave "sage tea" to "dry up" or reduce the amount of milk in mothers. They also used sage to treat female sterility and as a douche in leucorrhea.

Some old timers used sage to treat liver complaints, and also used a sage wash to treat old age leg ulcers or "bad veins."

The Indians used sage tea and sage baths to reduce fever as back in time as they could remember. This is probably where the herbal users picked up this treatment. The Indians also used sage leaves to clean their teeth. They rubbed their teeth and gums with the green sage leave.

Sage was used with other herbs to aid sleep an as a treatment of the flu.

Backwoods people made a tea from a handful of sage leaves and a handful of corn silk as a treatment for the kidneys and to "force" the water from the system.

Sage is chiefly composed of thujone and cineol. It also contains volatile oil (to 2%), tannins, oestrogens, organic acids, rosmarinic acid and bitter compounds including picrosalvine.

SAFFRON CROCUS (Crocus sativus)

The saffron crocus is found only as a yard flower today. At one time, it was used by herbalist to dye and perfume their herbal brews. The folks would be more likely to take a herbal medicine that looked good, instead of the normal brown, black, or green of the un-colored brews.

People used the saffron crocus to bring out the rash in small-pox, measles, scarlet fever, and other eruptive diseases.

Some said it would make "dry kidneys put out more water."

Saffron crocus contains oil (10%), essential oil; a bitter glycoside, picrocrocin; crocin, the glycoside of the coloring matter crocetin.

Saffron crocus had to be grown in the garden in the herbal period, so it was seldom used. For some reason, the rural folks expected the other people to have any hard to get herb when they needed it.

SASSAFRAS (Sassafras albidum)

Sassafras is the best known of the medical herbal plants. (tree) Its value as a healing herb is very limited and most people just considered it, more or less, a poor man's drink. It is now under scrutiny for possible toxicity problems. In fact, in many countries, sassafras had been withdrawn as a food flavoring.

The leaves of the sassafras were dried green (they still do) and ground into a powder for use in seasoning meats. In Southern regions of Louisiana, this sassafras powder is called "file" and used commonly in cooking "file gumbo."

Sassafras (root wood, root bark) was used as an aromatic, carminative, stimulant, diaphoretic and diuretic.

The country folks made a strong decoction by boiling the root bark and wood of the sassafras for about thirty minutes. Water was added to some of the decoction to make a tea weak enough to suit a given taste. They would force their children to drink the tea, believing it would build up their "blood." Some people developed a taste for the tea; however, most disliked the taste.

An infusion of sassafras was made by adding about a handful of root bark to a quart of boiling water. This is the safe way as little or none of the oil is released. This infusion had to be given over a long period of time in the treatment of rheumatism to show any results, if any.

Very knowledgeable herbalists soaked the pith of the sassafras in rain water and used it as an eye wash for inflammations of the eye.

Sassafras could be call a true "faith" herb, as there isn't anything in this herb to cure anything, except kill lice.

The old timers made a decoction of the inner bark and used the decoction for gastro-intestinal complaints. They also added the sassafras decoction to other medical herbs as a treatment for constipation.

The sassafras tree is considered by many authorities to have provided the first of the American medicinal plant drugs to reach Europe in 1564.

Sassafras contains: oil (to 3%), comprising safrole (to 80%), phellandrene and pinene. The oil of the sassafras was used to flavor tobacco and destroy lice.

News, movies and the T.V. Media glorified sassafras over the years. City reared children, when visiting their grandparents in the country, would ask their grandma to make them some sassafras tea. Over the years, these children and their children began to believe sassafras tea was a way of life in the country. Sassafras tea was seldom ever made in the normal living of the country people.

Warning: The oil of sassafras should not be used internally as it will damage the liver and kidney.

A few of the rural ladies, a little on the heavy side, swear they keep their weight down by drinking sassafras tea. They make an infusion from the bark of the sassafras roots. It was made by adding two handfuls of root bark to about a quart of water. It was boiled about thirty minutes. The dosage was a cup of the sassafras tea ever time they felt hunger. Some women said chewing a small limb of the sassafras tree would retard hunger.

Many of the rural women carried small twigs of sassafras and "chewed them to hide bad breath."

SAW PALMETTO (Serenoa Repens)

Most everyone has see the fan shaped leaves of the palmetto while driving through the country side in low areas. The Indians ground up the seed (fruit) and ate them as food. The Indians also believed the palmetto was a sedative and tonic.

The palmetto (partly dried ripe fruit) was used as a tonic, stimulant, expectorant, nutritive and sedative.

Some folks said the fruit has a local stimulant action on the mucous membranes of the respiratory and genito-urinary systems. They also used the palmetto fruit to treat cystitis, catarrh, bronchitis and as a tonic tea.

Some herbal quacks sold the palmetto fruit as a cure for sexual debility and atrophy of the testes, but I am inclined to believe this comes under the heading of "old wives tales." The Saw palmetto is very rare in some areas. They probably had to get it from the "root" man.

The saw palmetto contains: fixed oil (to 1.5%) to which the action is attributed.

SNEEZEWORT (Helenium autumnale)

The sneezewort (False sunflower/Sneezeweed) had but one purpose as herbal medicine. The whole plant was ground into a very fine powder. The powder was used as an errhine (snuff) to produce prolonged sneezing. The snuff was used to ease some headaches, fresh colds and some catarrhal complaints.

The folks claimed that religious fanatics would come to a dance and sprinkle the sneezewort powder on the floor to break up a dance.

SENECA SNAKE ROOT (Polygala senega) (Mountain Flax/Milkwort)

The root of the seneca snake root was one of the herbs that all folk medicine users dried and had on hand at all times.

Seneca snake root is a top of the line expectorant and all herbal users put great faith in its power. The seneca snake root is an energetic stimulant to the lungs.

Rural folks considered the seneca snake root a very valuable treatment in the advanced stages of chronic bronchitis, and "stubborn" whooping cough.

Most of the mothers used snake root to treat croup and bronchitis in infants and children.

The dosage of the powdered seneca snake root is two pinches mixed with syrup, milk or spirits.

A decoction was made from the root by simmering a small handful of the mashed root in a pint of boiling water. The keep a lid over the pot and simmered until about a third of a pint remains. Strain the liquid off. The dosage is about a third of a cup.

SLIPPERY ELM (Ulmus rubra)

Indians have long used the bark tea as both a laxative and as treatment for diarrhea. They also used the root tea to assist childbirth.

Slippery elm (dried powdered inner bark) was used as

a demulcent and emollient.

People used the dried inner bark of the slippery elm and ground it into a powder. They used the powder in the form of a poultice externally to treat ulcers, tumors, gunshot wounds, frost bite, burns, skin diseases, erysipelas, felons, etc. They mixed the powder in water and used it as a mouthwash to treat sore mouth or thrush.

Rural folks gave the slippery elm powder with water as a drink for consumptive patients and those who were recovering from an illness.

The inner bark of the slippery elm was at one time, used as a mechanical abortive so it is now only available commercially in the powdered, and, hence, harmless form.

Slippery elm contains mucilage, on hydrolysis yielding 3-methyl galactose.

SMARTWEED (Polygonum punctatum)

The smartweed (Biting knot weed/Water pepper) must be made in cold infusion. It only use in herbal medicine was in the treatment of suppressed menstruation. The dosage was to drink freely of the infusion for about a week. The dosage for a tincture of smartweed was a teaspoon three times a day.

STRAWBERRY (Fragaria vesca)

The strawberry, at one time, was believed to have many valuable medicinal properties. The prime use of the strawberry was to treat complaints of the bladder and kidneys.

The strawberry (fresh fruit, leaves, roots) was used as

an: astringent, diuretic, anti-scorbutic, tonic and laxative.

Herbal users made a decoction from the strawberry root and used the decoction to treat gonorrhea. They also gave the strawberry decoction as a diuretic and sometimes as a bitter tonic. The fruit was used as a laxative.

The strawberry contains (leaves) tannins, flavonoids; (fruit) organic acids, Vitamin C, mucilage and sugars.

The dried strawberry leaves were used as a substitute for tea in hard times.

SELF HEAL (Prunella vulgaris)

The self heal (Heal all/Woundwort) was used most often to stop the flow of blood in accidents and fights. The dried flowering plant was made into a strong infusion for most treatments. The powdered herb was used to stop bleeding by pouring it on the wound.

They used the self heal herb as a gargle or mouthwash to treat sore throat and any other inflammation of the mouth. It was also used to treat external ulcers, cuts, burns, wounds and bruises.

The rural herbal users, at one time, treated diphtheria with the self heal, although it was seldom used internally with the exception of mild diarrhea or flatulence.

They used the self heal as a bitter tonic and kept small bags of the powdered herb to stop bleeding.

The self heal contains volatile oil; tannins; an alkaloid; bitter principle and unknown substances.

SUMACH (Rhus Glabra)
(shoe-make)

Many old timers made an infusion of the sumach berries, sweetened with honey, as a gargle for sore throat.

Folks made an infusion of sumach berries, sweetened with sugar, as a treatment for diarrhea, dysentery and bowel complaints. They used the sumach bark to make a poultice to treat ulcers and old sores.

Herbal advocates made a decoction from the sumach bark and berries for suppression or incontinence of urine. The dosage was ten to fifteen drops of the decoction each day.

Some folks claim a decoction of the bark of the sumach root was used a wash in venereal and scrofulous diseases. Its exact use could not be determined.

Sumach was probably used when herbs for the same complaint were not available.

TOBACCO (Nicotiana Tabacum)

The country folks grew their little patches of tobacco for family use for years until "Big Brother" (feds) stepped in to stop it. (lost taxes) Tobacco contains nicotine which is very poisonous and one of the strongest poisons known.

The old timers mixed tobacco, mullein and jimson weed and smoked the mixture as a relief of asthma.

Folks blew smoke from tobacco into the ear to ease the pain of earache.

Tobacco juice was used on bites, insect stings and nettle stings.

I could not find any reliable information on tobacco

being used internally as medicine. Most old timers said they smoked tobacco because it was relaxing.

Blackleaf 40, a deadly poison is made from tobacco. It was used years back to kill pest in the garden or fields.

VIRGINIA SNAKEROOT (Aristolochia serpentaria)

(Birthwort/Serpentary)

Herbal users say that Virginia snakeroot will give protection from poisoning. The few herbal folds, who said they used this herb, claim it is very good for rattlesnake and mad-dog bites. With the knowledge of today, I do not think this could be true. If you get bitten by a rattlesnake or rabid dog, you better get to a doctor or hospital fast.

A few folks used the Virginia snakeroot to treat the early stages of some infectious diseases. One older man said he used it to perk up his appetite. This herb is seldom used in many areas.

The correct dosage has not been determined by herbalist. Virginia snakeroot could cause vomiting, vertigo and respiratory paralysis.

BETHROOT (Trillium sessile)

The bethroot (Squawroot/Wakerobin) genus consists of over twenty species. Some of the species are more effective than others. The bethroot was used primarily in the treatment of female complaints by Indians and early settlers. This herb has a fishy odor.

An infusion was made by adding a tablespoonful of the powdered bethroot (root) to a pint of boiling water. The dosage was determined by effect. Sometimes a teaspoonful of the powdered toot was given as a dose. The bethroot was also mixed with other herbs in some treatments.

Midwives used the bethroot for all problems before, during, and after childbirth where hemorrhages may occur.

Folks made a strong infusion by adding powdered bethroot to raspberry leaf tea. The dosage was two tablespoonfuls for the treatment of hemorrhages. This dosage was increased as required.

Rural users made a poultice of bethroot and blood root to treat tumors, carbuncles, ulcers, and other external sores.

Many of the rural hunters claimed that chewing the bethroot and swallowing the juice would cure the bit of the rattlesnake. Don't you ever believe this.

A few rural women used the bethroot juice in the treatment of long-time skin problems.

The bethroot was used in many other complaints where astringent action would be required.

The bethroot contains gum; tannin; volatile oil; fixed oil; and a saponin, trillarin.

This book is a history of how herbal medicine was used. This does not mean that a given treatment will, or will not work.

WATERCRESS (Nasturtium officinale)

Watercress is so common that most herbal have forgotten that it is a very good medical herb. The pungency of this herb discourages many from using it. Some people like the taste of watercress.

Watercress contains Vitamins A, B2, C, D, E; nicotinamide; a glucoside, gluconasturtin; volatile oil comprising phenylethlisothiocyanate; minerals including iron, manganese, phosphorus, iodine and calcium.

Watercress is mixed with honey and used as a cough remedy. A handful of watercress is steeped (infusion) in a cup of water and the liquid drained off. This liquid is added to the honey to make a cough syrup.

In a few areas, watercress is used to treat asthma. It is also used as a purgative when more active herbs are not available.

Some folks claim watercress was used as an aphrodisiac and contraceptive. One would be inclined to list this under the same category as the manure cures, no basic for the claims.

Watercress can be eaten raw, cooked as greens or made into a soup. Most people just do not like the taste of watercress.

WILD-GINGER (Hexastylis arifolla)

A tea was made from the wild-ginger. (Jug-plant) It was used for the treatment of flatulence and colic. A snuff was made from the root to relieve headaches. The tea was used for indigestion.

Wild-ginger contains volatile oil; a bitter principle; resin; asarin; alkaloid and sugars. Some folks called the wild-ginger a female herb. They did not say how it was used on female complaints.

WATERMELON (Citrullus rulgaris)

The old timers gave copious amounts of watermelon to treat several different kidney complaints. I was unable to get more accurate details.

Farmers painted watermelons with a lime white wash so that the melons would keep for some time. Others made preserves of the watermelon rinds and used them for food and medical treatment.

The younger ladies in rural areas mixed watermelon and cucumber into a mush. They covered their face with the mush as a cleaner.

There is a kidney ailment that to this day can be treated only by watermelon juice.

WORMWOOD (Artemisia absinthium)

Wormwood (Absinthe/Green ginger) was better known by the rural folks who operated "white lightning" stills many years back. They would take the best "drippings" for their own use. An infusion of wormwood would be added to the remainder of a given batch. This would be sold to "outsiders." This would give the white lightening the kick of a mule. White lightening laced with wormwood was one of the strongest and most dangerous "corn lickens."

Folks prepared wormwood as a powder and an infusion. A dose of the powder was just a pinch. A handful of the wormwood was added to a quart of cold water to make an infusion. The dosage of the infusion was one tablespoonful. It was used as a stimulant and tonic by many folks to treat dyspepsia, diarrhea, and worms.

Herbalists, in some areas, used the wormwood to treat hysteria, epilepsy, neuralgia, and other nervous complaints.

Wormwood is very dangerous. It contains bitter principle, volatile oil, a glucoside, resins, starch and santonin.

The plant called "rabbit tobacco" in some areas may be wormwood.

WHITE OAK (Quercus alba)

Not many white oaks remain in many areas, as over the years, nearly all the white oaks have been cut for lumber.

The white oak bark is very astringent. The bark of the young branches was used by nearly all herbal users.

A decoction was made from the bark of the white oak and used external as a wash for gangrenous ulcers and other sores and wounds.

Midwives injected the white oak decoction to treat the falling of the womb or bowels.

Many folks made a decoction of roasted white oak acorns. This was given as a remedy for diarrhea, dyspepsia and scrofula.

Although many books claim the white oak acorns was poison, many folks ate the acorns after they turned brown. Some people roasted them. I have ate many of a white oak acorn and suffered no known effect. It sure doesn't harm deer and hogs, etc. when they eat them.

WILD INDIGO (Baptisia SP.)

The information obtained on wild indigo week is all from the second person, such as, "Grandma said." This would indicated that wild indigo has not been active in herbal medicine for some time. Wild indigo is also known as the Horse-fly weed and yellow broom.

A decoction was made from the outer layer of the bark of the wild indigo. It was used in treating protracted fevers, such as typhus and typhoid. A decoction was also made by adding a handful of the fresh root to a quart of boiling water for internal use. The dosage was a tablespoonful every four hours. This decoction was used also as a wash to treat sores in the mouth.

A poultice was made from the wild indigo for external use on sores.

False indigo also grows near wild indigo. Should anyone use false indigo by mistake, somebody will long regret it. Wild indigo was grown to make dye in the 1800's.

WILD CHERRY

(Prunus virginiana & Prunus serotina)
(black cherry/Rum cherry

There are two wild cherries listed. The Wild cherry grows in most of the South.

The bark of the root or trunk is ground into a powder and soaked in cold water for two or three days. Hot water will destroy the healing power of the bark. The dosage is about half a cup three times a day.

Herbal users gave the cold wild cherry bark infusion for many complaints such as fevers, consumption, dysentery, chronic diarrhea, colic, debility, dyspepsia and most all complaints of the stomach.

The old folks made syrup from the powdered black cherry bark to treat colds and irritating coughs. Black cherry bark is still used by pharmacopoeia for the same purpose.

The fruit and dried fruit stalks were used as a diuretic and astringent.

The black cherry fruit stalks contains tannic acid, potassium salts and flavonoids. The fruit contains organic acid, provitamin A and tannin.

Warning: The leaves of the wild cherry contain cyanide at some stage during their growth.

Herbal users said, "Never give wild cherry for a dry cough." They never gave the reason why.

Many of the rural folks claim wild cherry tea made from the ground bark would keep "heart pressure down."

The Wild cherry must be made by cold infusions.

COMMON WILLOW (Salix Alba or S. Nigra)

Over one hundred different types of the willow grows in the United States. The Indians and later, settlers chewed the leaves of the willow tree to relieve a headache. Whether one or all of the willow tree leaves will give this relief is not known. There is some question as to what part of the willow really was used.

Nearly all herbal users made a decoction from the bark of the willow tree and used it for the treatment of headaches.

Salicin, the active ingredient in the willow bark is the basis for aspirin; therefore, this would indicate that the bark was used.

WHITE WATER LILY (Nymphaea odorata)

There is some question as to which water lily was used in a given area. There is the white water lily and the white pond lily. They may be the same.

The white water lily contains alkaloids, especially nupharine; tannins as nymphea-tannic acid; a cardenolide, nymphanine; mucilage.

One old man said his family made a decoction from the water lily. They used it as a gargle for sore throat, to wash external sores, and, during hard times, as a soap.

A herbal user said a tea from the water was used to slow down the heart beat. He also claimed it would improve sex drive.

One very old women said she gave her husband water lily tea all the time to "slow his demands." This shows that you need many more users to determine the facts about a given herb.

WITCH HAZEL (Hamamelis virginiana)

The witch hazel blooms in the winter after the leaves fall, so you will not have a problem locating the witch hazel.

The witch hazel (bark, leaves, flower-bearing twigs) was used for an astringent and hemostatic.

The old timers made an infusion for the witch hazel leaves to treat or stop hemorrhages of the rectum, nose and uterus; also to treat hemorrhoids and varicose vein.

A tincture was made from the witch hazel and added to other herbs in the treatment of typhoid fever and some "sturburn" cases of diarrhea.

A diluted tincture of witch hazel was applied to bruises and sprains to give relief.

The witch hazed contains tannin, comprising hamomelitannin (bark 6%); leaves (12%), gallic acid, calcium oxalate, traces of volatile oil, saponin and flavonoids pigments. The leaves also contain phlobatannin.

Caution: modern distilled witch hazel is extremely astringent and may damage the skin unless diluted.

WHITE SNAKE ROOT (Eupatorium rugosum)
(white sanicle/Pool root)

A handful of the bruised root was placed in a pint of boiling water to make an infusion of the white snake root. The dosage was from one to four tablespoonfuls of the infusion. A very limited number of folks used this herb in the lower South.

The infusion was used to treat the "all overs" and other nervous complaints. It was also used to treat Pleurisy and convulsions. It was used to treat nearly all lung complaints.

YARROW (Achillea millefollum)
(Woundwort/Milfoul)

The yarrow plant was used in the treatment of wounds since ancient times. An infusion of the yarrow plant (dried plant, less roots) was made by adding a cup of the herb to a pint of water and reducing by heat to a half pint. The dosage was a tablespoonful every hour. The juice from the yarrow plant was given three times a day. The dosage was three tablespoonfuls.

The nearest medical terms to describe its use in herbal medicine would be diaphoretic, antipyretic, hypotensive and diuretic.

The rural users gave yarrow for the "runs," gripes and bloody-fluxes." They mixed the yarrow with elder flowers to treat colds and the flu. Many said the fresh leaves would "kill toothache."

The young rural girls mixed yarrow and cucumber juice to clean "greasy skin."

Midwives used yarrow to treat piles, leucorrhea, menorrhagia, amenorhea, dyspepsia and flatulent colic. They also used yarrow to regulate menstrual periods.

Many old folks said yarrow was good for "strokes." They also claimed to put powdered yarrow in their snuff to prevent strokes.

Some used yarrow juice to clean wounds and to slow bleeding.

Yarrow was a tonic to treat "sour craw" and other like ailments.

The yarrow plant contains volatile oil containing azuiene; and a glycoalkaloid, achillein. Large doses of yarrow will cause headaches and vertigo.

YELLOW JESSAMINE (Gelsemium sempervirens)

(Yeller Jesum)

Only a very few knowledgeable herbalists ever attempted to use the "yeller Jesum" (Yellow jessamine) in herbal medicine.

The yellow jessamine (dried rhizome and root) was used as a sedative and nervine.

The expert herbal users used the yellow jessamine for the treatment of sick headaches, neuralgia, menstrual and rheumatic pains and migraine. I could not find out in what manner the yellow jessamine was prepared for use as a medicine.

Most herbal users would not use the yellow jessamine for any type of treatment.

The yellow jessamine contains alkaloids; gelsemine, sempervirine and gelsemicine, phytosterol, resin, fixed oil, emodin monomethylether ether and methylacculetin.

DANGER: All parts of the yellow jessamine are poisonous. the toxic effects include double vision, giddiness, respiratory depression and DEATH. Gelsemium is more strongly depressant than hemlock.

YELLOW LADY'S-SLIPPER

(Cypripedium calceolus)

The yellow lady's-slipper is closely related to pubescens. Very little use of the lady's-slipper was indicated by herbal users.

The root was used in the treatment of hysteria, insomnia and nervous headaches. This plant may cause hallucinations. The rural folks say this plant will make the skin "burn bad."

The yellow lady's-slipper contains volatile oils; two resins; glucosides; tannin and gallic acid.

This plant in now rare and should not be destroyed.

HERBAL CLAIMS

This is a list of herbs the herbal users claim to have healing power. Some of them are valid. Some are very dangerous, and many of these claims come under quackery. They are listed for your information only.

You must remember that herbs contain real chemicals and drugs, good, bad, and ineffective. Would you go into a drug store and start using any drug you find there? Well, the same applies to herbs.

ALFALFA: Buffalo herb, lucerne

Alfalfa is a rich sub-nutritional food with trace minerals and has some value in herbal medicine. Alfalfa is said to cure or treat: Diabetes, TB, rheumatism, Bright's disease, toxemia, jaundice, neuralgia, insomnia, nervousness, syphilis, constipation, lumbago, hardening of the arteries, dropsy, prostititis, anemia, skin eruption, poor complexion, teeth, bones, inflamed bladder, removes poison from the body, and produces milk for nursing mothers. If all of the above claims were true, this would be the only herb you would ever need.

ALOES: Aloes Vera Aloe Socotrain

Herbalists claim aloes will cure or treat: Burns, bruises, clean the colon, expel worms, promote menstruation, cleans the stomach, liver kidneys, spleen, bladder, clears throat. You better just stick to burns, cuts, and bruises when using aloes. Do not use if pregnant.

Althea: Althea officinalis, Marrow Family, Marshmallow

Herbalist use althea root to treat or cure; Inflamed eyes, irritation of the vagina, diarrhea, dysentery, inflamed bladder, kidneys and mucous membranes.

ANGELICA: Angelica Atropurpurea, archangel

Angelica roots and seed were used by herbalist to cure or treat: Stomach trouble, gas, colic, heartburn, cold, fever, and deafness. It is further claimed to stop poisons, and inhibit the drinking of liquors.

ANISE: Pimpinella anisum

Herbalist used anise seed to treat or cure: colic, nausea, prevent gas in the stomach and bowels, aids digestion and relieves over-eating.

ANNOTTO: Achitoe

Annatto seed contains a large amount of Vitamin A and D.

ARNICA: Arnica montana, Leopard's Bane

Folks used arnica flowers in liniments for strains, bruises, sprains, pain, muscular rheumatism.

ASPARAGUS: Asparagus officinale

Asparagus is an outstanding food for any table. Herbalist used asparagus to treat kidney and bladder stones, dropsy, and as a heart sedative. It is a diuretic, so these claims may be true. Some say it will keep old folks from becoming senile.

BALM OF GILEAD: populus balsamifea

Balm of gilead buds must be boiled in oil to make an ointment or salve. Folks used balm of gilead to treat colds, lungs, kidneys and urinary problems.

BASIL: Ocium Basilicum

Folk medicine people used basil leaves to treat suppressed menstruation, vomiting, expels afterbirth, and claimed to be effective on snake bites and insect stings.

BLACK COHOSH: Cimicifuga racemosa

Black cohosh root is claimed by folks to treat or cure: The nervous system, epilepsy, convulsions, acute rheumatism, neuralgia, spinal meningitis, snake-bite poisoning, start menstrual flow, high blood pressure, and whooping cough.

BLACK HAW: Cimicifuga racemosa

People used the black haw root bark to treat: Threatened abortion, after pains asthma, hysteria, and used in female tonics.

BLUE COHOSH: Viburnum rufidulum

Folks used the blue cohosh root to treat or cure: Uterine disorders, epilepsy, cramps, dropsy, colic, hysteria, high blood pressure, and diabetes.

BLUE FLAG: Iris versicolour

The blue flag rhizome was used by folks to treat: Thyroid gland, diuretic, vermifuge, and other vague claims.

BONESET: Eupatorium perioliatium

Herbalists used the boneset tops and leaves to treat debility, typhoid fever, general influenza, and to produce perspiration. It was also used as a laxative and a tonic. You will notice that is about the most bitter herb around.

BORAGE: Borago officinalis

Borage is said to expel poisons, comforts the heart form grief, good for mother's milk, sore eyes and hepatitis.

BURDOCK: Arctium lappa

Burdock root is believed to be blood purifier, will remove or treat all skin diseases, carbuncles and boils, eruptions, burns, wounds, and hemorrhoids. Burdock also is said to be good for sciatica, leprosy, inflammation, bruises, sprains, and many other superfluous maladies.

CAMOMILE: Anthemis nobills

Camomile flowers made into a tonic are used to treat

quinsy, stomach, gas digestion, colic in infants, typhoid fever, and will produce perspiration. A poultice of Camomile is said to prevent gangrene and also removes any gangrenous tissue.

CARAWAY: Carum carui

Caraway seed are use to treat colic in infants, aid the stomach, good for female troubles, remove black and blue spots of bruises. Some people say they eat the roots like parsnips

CASCARA SAGRADA: Rhamunus purschians

Cascara sagrada is an Indian remedy for constipation. It is not much used by other people.

CATNIP: Nepeta cataria

See catnip in this book.

CAYENNE: Capsicum annum

See cayenne in this book. Cayenne is said to be a strong stimulant, and is also used in the treatment of debility, indigestion, chills, heart failure, and costiveness. Cayenne is also used for coughs, colds, quincy, diphtheria, scarlet fever, sore throat , and asthma. Cayenne is given often and in small doses. It is truly effective for some of the above ailments.

CELERY: Apium Graveolens

Herbalists used the celery roots and seed as a tonic to regulate urine. Treat dropsy, liver troubles, nervousness, neuralgia, and rheumatism

CHESTNUT: Castamoa

Chestnut leaves were used to treat hiccoughs and coughs.

CHICKWEED: Stellaria Media

Folks used the leaves of the chickweed to treat: Pleurisy, bronchitis, colds, coughs, rheumatism, hoarseness, inflammation of the bowels or stomach. External treatments includes skin diseases, boils, sore eyes, burns, tumors, erysipelas, hemorrhoids, obesity, and sore throat.

CHICORY: Cichorium endiva

See chicory in the book. The chicory root was used by folks to treat the kidneys, liver, stomach, spleen, and jaundice. Drink chicory with your coffee.

CLEAVERS: Galium aparine

Herbalists used the whole herb to cure or treat ailments. It is used to clear the skin, as a blood cleaner, remove bladder stones, stop bleeding, as a reducing aid. It is also used to treat: Dropsy, scarlet fever, eczema, measles, jaundice, old sores, and summer complaints.

Remember that all the ailments listed in this HERBAL CLAIMS section are what the herbalists claim they will cure or treat and in no ways means that the herbs will.

COLOMBO: Cocculus palmatus

Colombo is a bitter tonic and may aid some complaints. Herbal people used it to treat fevers, colon troubles, diarrhea, cholera, and to stop vomiting.

COLTS FOOT: Tussilago farfara

Colts foot roots and leaves are used in the treatment of sinusitis, asthma, bronchitis, coughs, whooping cough and fevers. Most people used it in the form of a cough syrup.

COMFREY: Symphytum officinale

See comfrey in this book. The roots and leaves of the comfrey were used by folks as a remedy for coughs, sinusitis, lung trouble, asthma, kidneys, stomach, or bowels, bloody urine, bruises, sprains, fractures, burns, gangrene, and ulcers. Poultices, teas and salves were the most common method of use.

CORIANDER: Coriandrum satium

Coriander seed was used as a stomach tonic, laxative, and purgative to expel gas from the bowels.

CORN SILK. Stigmata maidis, Zea Mays

Used as a strong tea. It was used to treat: irritable conditions of the urinary organs, bed wetting, bladder, kidney and prostate ailments.

CREEPING JENNY: European bindweed.

Creeping jenny roots were used to stop bleeding upon contact with wound.

DANDELION: Taraxicum dens-leonis

See dandelion this book. The leaves and roots were used to treat or cure jaundice, eczema, kidney troubles, inflammation of the bowels, fever, female organ, liver, pancreas, spleen, and uterine obstructions.

DILL Anethum graveolens

See dill this book. Dill seed was used to control the nerves, stop hiccoughs, quicken the brain, and expel gas and other vague claims.

ELECAMPANE: inula helenium

People used the roots of elecampane to treat whooping cough, gastric membranes, retention of urine, delayed menstruation, kidney or bladder stones, and liver. It is an expectorant.

ELDERBERRY: Sambucus

See elderberry in this book. The elderberry is used to treat erysipelas, dropsy, burns, scalds, pneumonia, and complexion disorders. It contains a fair amount of Vitamin C.

EYEBRIGHT: Euphrasia officinale

Herbalists used eyebright leaves to treat coughs, earaches, and sinusitis. Some claim it will restore sight and memory. Better think about these claims.

FENNEL: Foeniculum officinale

See fennel this book. Fennel was used to treat or cure: acid stomach, cramps and colic in infants, obesity, increases menstrual flow, hiccoughs, and will increase milk flow in mothers.

FLEABANE: Ergeron caradense

Herbalists used the whole plant in their treatments. It was used to treat summer complaint, all overs, colon trouble, bladder, scalding urine, hemorrhages of the bowels or uterus. It was also used an enema.

GENTIAN: Gentiana lutea

The root of the gentian was used in folk medicine. Gentian was used in or as a treatment for blood, liver, fevers, colds, for scanty urine, malarial, suppressed menstruation, and chills. They also claimed it allays poison from mad-dog bites, insect and snake bites. They claim gentian acts like quinine.

GINSENG: Panax quinquefolia

The ginseng root is used in herbal medicine. Herbal users say it is good for the appetite, digestive disturbances, colds, chest troubles, coughs, constipation, inflammation of urinary tract and to increase sex drive.

GOLDEN SEAL: Hydrastix candadensis

The roots of golden seal are use in herbal medicine. Golden seal was used to treat colds, stomach, liver, sores, eczema, erysipelas, ringworm, skin disease, nausea, tonsils, spinal meningitis, scarlet fever, smallpox, pyorreha, typhoid fever, spleen, and diphtheria.

HOPS: Humulus Lupulus

The cones of the hops were used in folk medicine. Hops was used to treat sleeplessness, coughs, abscesses, delirium tremens, all-overs, toothache, liver, urine flow, boils, tumors, ulcers, after-pains, and bronchitis. It was also used for diseases of the throat and chest. Hops is a nervine.

HOREHOUND: Marrubium vulgare

The whole plant was used. It was used for perspiration, as a laxative, jaundice, asthma, hysteria, to expel worms, coughs, sore throat, control menstruation flow, croup, to expel afterbirth, to eliminate poisons, and to clear the vision. Remember, these are only claims.

HORSEMINT: Monarda Punctata

The leaves and tops were used to treat athlete's foot, psoriasis, and impetigo.

HYSSOP: Hyssopus officinalis

The whole plant of the hyssop was used. The hyssop was used to increase circulation, reduce blood pressure, kill body and hair lice, expel worms, reduce fever, as an eye wash, for treating quinsy. It was also used to treat sore throat, asthma, coughs, and spasms in infants. This is a Biblical remedy, so be careful what you say around rural folks.

JUNIPER: Juniperus communis

See juniper in this book. The bark and berries were used in folk medicine.

LADY SLIPPER: Cypridedium Pubescens

Folks used the root to treat hysteria, nervous irritablity, and nervous headache.

LIQUORICE: Glycirrhiza glabra

The root was used most times for coughs and as an laxative.

LILY OF THE VALLEY: Convallaria majalis

The roots of the lily of the valley was used to treat epilepsy, dropsy, convulsions, dizziness, palsy, all-overs, and apoplexy. They claim it will also make your brain brighter, and will quite the heart.

LOBELIA: Lobelia inflata

See lobelia this book. Herbalist say lobelia does not cure much alone, but is effective when combined with other herbs. It is a powerful relaxant. It was used to treat pleurisy, whooping cough, hepatitis, angina pectorals, laryngitis, scarlet fever, chicken pox, measles, small pox, diphtheria, lock-jaw, asthma, all-overs, and other complaints.

MANDRAKE: Podophyllum pelatum (May Apple)

See mandrake this book. Herbalist used the root of the mandrake internally and externally to treat cancers, ulcers, wounds, amenorrhea, and hepatitis. It was also used for bruises, sprains, smallpox and measles, Mandrake is a very powerful bowel regulator, or un-regulator, so you better take heed.

MARIGOLD: Calendula

See marigold this book. This is one of the better herbs and you should take time to investigate it.

MARJORAM: Origanum marhorana

The whole plant was use as atonic or poultice. They used it to treat sprains, felons, boils, carbuncles, loss of appetite, suppressed menstruation, hepatitis, deafness, headache, indigestion, nausea, colic neuralgia, toothache, and other complaints. It was also used to expel poisons.

MILKWEED: Asclepias syriaca

See milkweed this book. Herbalists used the milkweed to treat female troubles, kidney and bowel trouble, dropsy, asthma, stomach trouble, and to remove gallstones.

MISTLETOE: Viscum flavescens

See mistletoe this book. It is a narcotic and nervine. This is a very dangerous herb. Better take notice.

MOTHERWORT: Leonurus cardiaca

The tops and leaves of the motherwort were used in herbal medicine. It is a laxative and a nervine, so you better use with care. It was used to treat (Treat, cure, sure cure, does not have a real meaning in herbal and folk medicine) female troubles, cramps, hysteria, convulsions, sleeplessness, delirium tremens, liver disorders, suppressed urine, colds, and to increase menstrual flow. They say it will expel worms and strengthen the heart.

MULLEIN: Verbascum thapsus

See mullein this book. The roots, leaves and flowers were used in folk medicine. Mullein was used in the form of a tea, fermentation, poultice, ointment, syrup, tincture and the leaves were also used just as they came from the plant. The roots were burnt and the fumes were inhaled in some treatments. Fresh crushed flowers was claimed to remove warts. Mullein was used to treat asthma, croup, bronchitis, all lung ailments, bleeding from the lungs, difficult breathing, hay fever, and as a gargle. It was used to induce sleep and to relieve pain. Mullein was also used to treat sinusitis, swollen joints, dropsy, diarrhea, prostate swelling, bad sores, coughs, sciatica, rheumatism, spinal soreness, neuralgia, hemorrhoids, and mumps. Many of the above claims are valid and just as many are questionable. People, as a rule, were lazy and mullein being close at hand in all areas, was the reason it was used in so many treatments.

MYRRH: Balsamodendron myrrh

A powdered gum from the myrrh was used in herbal medicine. It was used to treat bronchial and lung diseases, halitosis, sick stomach, hemorrhoids, gangrene, coughs, asthma, chest complaints, mucous discharges, and toothaches. It was also used to treat shock, collapse and prostration.

NETTLE: Urtica Dioca, Stinging Nettle.

See nettle in this book. The leaves and roots of the nettle was used to treat kidney trouble, bladder stones, flow of urine, diarrhea, worms, dropsy, hemorrhaging from urinary organs, lungs, intestines, stomach and nose. It was also used as a blood purifier, shampoo, phlegm remover, menstrual control, treatment for summer complaint. A man even claimed he grew a third set of molars by eating nettle leave. Would you really believe nettle will do all the above claims? I sure hope not.

PAPAYA: Tropical fruit

Papaya was used to treat stomach and bowel complaints.

PARSLEY: Petroselinum sativum

They roots, leaves and seed of parsley was used in herbal medicine. Parsley was used to treat hepatitis, fevers, difficult urination, obstruction of spleen and liver, female troubles, insect bites and stings, swollen glands, swollen breasts, scarlantina, and dropsy.

PEACH: Amygdalus persica

See peach in this book. The peach roots, leaves, twigs, and kernels were used in treatments. They were used to treat whooping cough, hepatitis, worms, nausea, bladder and uterine complaints, vomiting, in cholera morbus, sores, baldness and other complaints. Peach leaves were sometimes used instead of quinine. Don't use the peach kernel in treatments as only your relatives will know you made a mistake.

PENNYROYAL: Hedeoma Pulegioides

The whole pennyroyal plant was used to treat fevers, chest, lungs, leprosy, dropsy, hepatitis, colic, headache, cramps, nausea, bruises, black eyes, nervousness, hysterics, spasms, TB, coughs, and whooping coughs.. Pennyroyal was also used to ward off mosquitoes.

PEPPERMINT: Mentha piperita

People used peppermint to treat fevers, chills, gas on stomach, vomiting, nausea, diarrhea, cholera, heart trouble, colds and hysteria. It was also used to treat rheumatism, neuralgia, headache, toothache, colon trouble, convulsions, spasms, insanity fainting, dizzy spells, toothaches, and seasickness. I believe they are claiming too much for this herb. Bear in mind that some herbs was given just to give relief, not cure.

POKE WEED: Phytolacca decandra

See poke weed in this book. The roots leaves and

berries were used. The red stems was not used. The poke weed has many valid herbal treatments and is used today in modern medicine in the form of drugs. It is a wonder herb. This is a dangerous herb when misused.

PRICKLY ASH: Xanthoxylum

See prickly ash in this book. They used prickly ash to treat toothache, tongue, mouth, rheumatism, hepatitis, and mucous membranes. Prickly ash may cause vomiting.

ROSEMARY: Rosemarinu officinalis

The leaves and flowers of the rosemary were used as a remedy for colds, colic, nervous ailments, nervous headache, bad gums, halitosis, sore throat, insanity, indigestion, coughs, rheumatism, and arthritis.

RUE: Saliva officinalis

See rue in this book. Rue is a very dangerous herb and should be left to the herbal experts. It was used as a remedy for stomach, cramps, nervousness, hysteria, convulsions, dizziness, insanity, worms, headache, colic, sciatica, joint pain, gout, and other complaints. A tincture of the seed was used as an antidote fro deadly poisons.

SAGE: Saliva officinalis

See sage in this book. The sage leaves were used in herbal medicine. This is one of the outstanding herbs used in folk medicine. They used sage to treat nerves, palsy, quinsy, sore throat, worms, bleeding, kidney, liver, fevers, flu, headaches, dandruff, breasts and other complaints. Mother's breast feeding their baby should not use sage as it will dry up her milk.

SARSAPARILLA: Smilax officinalis

The root of the sarsaparilla is used. It was used as an antidote for deadly poisons. It was also used to increase the flow of urine, as an eyewash, promote perspiration, treat venereal disease in infants. Medical research has discovered that it contains organic hormones. Look out for the sex promoters!

SASSAFRAS: Laurua-Sassafras officinalis

See sassafras in this book. The bark, roots and leaves were used. This is an overrated herb of no rear value in herbal medicine except to kill lice. This is a faith herb and those who believe in it will get relief. They claim it will purify blood, relieve gas and colic, aid in kidney or bladder trouble. It may work as a diuretic and as a wash for sores.

SKULLCAP: Scutellaria Lateriflora

Skullcap is a nervine and should be used with caution. They used skullcap to treat heart weakness, nerves, hydrophobia, snake bites, delirium tremens, St. Vitus Dance, shaking palsy, lock-jaw, ague, fevers, and neuralgia. Better to leave this herb to those who know.

SHEPHERD'S PURSE: Capsella Bursa Pastoris

They used shepherd's purse to stop bleeding and hemorrhages of all kinds.

SLIPPERY ELM: Ulmua Fulva

See slippery elm in this book. The inter bark was used to treat dysentery, diarrhea, urinary tract, bronchitis, heartburn, inflammations, boils, sore throat, and other complaints. It was also used as a suppository, and an antidote for many poisons.

SORREL: Rumex acetosa

The roots and leaves were used to expel worms, expel kidney stones, and to treat hepatitis, boils, and tumors. Sorrel must be used while it is green.

SPEARMINT: Mentha viridis

The whole plant was used. It was used to treat colic, gas in the stomach and bowels, dropsy, nausea, bladder stones, kidneys and nerves.

SQUAW VINE: Mitchella Repens

The whole plant was used. Midwives used the squaw vine in childbirth. Folks used it to treat sore eyes, uterine troubles, female complaints, sore nipples, and skin sores.

SWEET BALM: Melissa officinalis

The whole plant was used. They used sweet balm to treat fevers, colds, flu, nausea, kidneys, bladder, headache, suppressed urine, painful menstruation, and female disorders.

VALERIAN: Valerina officinalis

The roots were used. This herb is a nervine and requires caution. It was used to treat hysteria, measles, scarlet fever, restlessness, colic, fevers, colds, gravel, coughs, shortness of breath, ease pain, and remove phlegm from the throat. It was also used as a sleep aid.

VIOLET: Clematis virginica

The leaves and flowers were used. They were used to

treat severe headache, ulcers, bad sores, and eruptive diseases.

WAHOO: Euonymus atropurpureus

The bark and roots were used in herbal medicine. The country folks used it to treat chest and lung ailments, torpid liver, fevers, pancreas, spleen, dropsy, digestion, chills, constipation, and pulmonary ailments.

WILD CHERRY: Purnus Virginiana

See wild cherry in this book. The bark and fruit of the wild cherry was used to treat T.B., bronchitis, fever, coughs, diarrhea, indigestion, asthma, colds, flu, and to reduce blood pressure. Do not boil wild cherry bark.

WILD PLUM:

The bark of the wild plum was used to treat asthma.

WINTERGREEN: Gaultheria Procumbens

The leaves of the wintergreen was used. It was used to stimulate stomach, heart and respiratory tract. It was also used to treat rheumatic fever, sciatica, bladder troubles, skin diseases, colic dropsy, cystitis, stomach, bowel obstructions, boils, swellings, ulcers, felons, leucorrhea, sore throat, and arthritis.

WITCH HAZEL: Hamamelis Virginica

See witch hazel in this book. The bark, twigs, and leaves were used. They used witch hazel to stop excessive menstruation, hemorrhages from the lungs, stomach, uterus and bowels. It as also used to treat diarrhea, nose bleed, and hemorrhoids. It was used as an enema and gargle.

YARROW: Achillea millefolium
Milfoil/Woundwort/Carpenter's Weed

The whole yarrow plant was used. It was used to control bleeding from the lungs. It was also used to treat or cure measles, chicken pox, smallpox, typhoid fever, diarrhea, colic, colds, uterine ailments, and leucorrhea, Yarrow contains a trace of sulphur.

Used as a (Dried plant and flowers, no roots) Diaphoretic; antipyretic; hypotensive; diuretic and urinary antiseptic.

YELLOW DOCK: Rumex crispus

The roots was used. It was used to treat eruptive diseases, swellings, leprosy, eyes, and blood.

Although many of the herbal plants listed under herbal claims are not native to all areas, many of the old folks came from areas where the herbs grew. Time and time again, they would say, "I could cure (a certain ailment) if only I had a (given) herb."

The herbal trade was fairly large at one time. Very little of its history was ever recorded. Few people of today ever heard of the root man or root stand where people could buy or trade herbs.

Herbal medicine is still used in many rural areas. The method of treatment will not vary much from place to place. Many of you are using herbal and folk medicine and don't even know it.

COMPLAINT AND HERBAL TREATMENT

ALCOHOL ABUSE

Angelica, cayenne pepper, chamomile, watercress.

ALLERGIES

Honey comb, apple cider vinegar, ginseng.

ANEMIA

Carrot juice.

ANTISEPTICS

Cabbage, carrot, cinnamon bark, clove, sweet clover, creosote bush, red currant, garlic, ginger, goldenseal, horse-radish, juniper, onions, radish, sage and thyme. Note: The antiseptics herbs above do work.

ARTHRITIS

Apple cider vinegar, ginger, burdock root.

ASTRINGENT HERBS.

Oak bark, bayberry bark, red raspberry, white poplar, witch hazel, yellow dock, cranesbill, wild geranium.

BED WETTING

Marjoram, mullein, St. John's wort, pumpkin seeds. Note: Nothing will work in young children until their bladder is fully developed. In some children, this may take years.

BITES

Banana, castor oil, clay, feverfew, garlic, marigold,

oat meal, onion, plantain, rue, wormwood.

BLEEDING AND CUTS

Cayenne pepper, juniper berries, lemon, marigold, puff ball, red raspberry, sanicle, shepherd's purse, okra.

BLISTERS

Peach pits.

BOILS AND ABSCESSES

Cabbage, fig, honey, onion, garlic, peach, radish, slippery elm, thyme.

BREASTS

Peach, parsley, peppermint

BRUISES

Agrimony, arnica, cabbage, caraway, comfrey, daisy, mullein, onion, shepherd's purse, Solomon's seal, vinegar, witch hazel, yarrow.

BURNS

Aloe vera, blueberry, potato water.

CHAPPED HANDS

Leak, oat meal, aloe vera.

CHILBLAIN (Frost bite)

Cayenne pepper, ginger, onion, potato.

COLDS

Anise, balm, barley water, borage, cinnamon, garlic,

ginseng, honey, lemon, peppermint, mustard, yarrow, chicken soup.

CONSTIPATION

Apple, clove, figs, honey, licorice, prunes, spinach, strawberry.

COUGHS-BRONCHITIS-ASTHMA

Almond, anise, camphor, wild cherry, coltsfoot, dock, elecampane, garlic, ginseng, honey, horehound, lemon, lime flowers, licorice, mullein, mustard, onion, pine tree, peppermint, slippery elm, wintergreen.

CRAMPS AND MUSCLE SPASMS

Arnica, peppermint, eucalyptus, vinegar.

CYSTITIS

Acidophilus, cranberry, garlic.

DETOXIFICATION

Apple pectin, basil, cloves, cayenne pepper, coffee, fennel, hay flowers, oat meal, oatstraw, peach, salt, baking soda.

DIARRHEA

Agrimony, barley, blackberry, lime flowers, nutmeg, peppermint, rice, yellow pond lily.

DIGESTIVE FLATULENCE AND INDIGESTION

Anise, caraway, cayenne pepper, centaury, chamomile, cinnamon, cloves, coriander, cumin, dill, fennel, ginger, juniper berries, nutmeg, peppermint, valerian.

DIURETIC

Apple, celery, corn silk, grapes, juniper, onions, parsley.

EARS

Caraway, chamomile, garlic, wild ginger, mullein, onions, yarrow.

ECZEMA

Aloe vera, blackberry leaf, oat meal, artichoke, elecampane.

EYES

Apple, borage, cabbage, chamomile, cucumber, eyebright, fennel, goldenseal, rose water, tansy, thyme, witch hazel, yarrow.

FELON

Lemon, garlic, onion, cabbage leaf.

FEVER

Apple, barley water, cayenne pepper, fenugreek, ginseng, grapes, lemon, raspberry vinegar, rice, strawberries.

FLU PREVENTION

Cayenne pepper, vinegar, salt, cinnamon, licorice.

GLANDS

Apple cider vinegar, burdock, cumin, fennel, flaxseed, ginseng.

HAIR TONICS

Apple cider vinegar, burdock, nettle, rhubarb, sage.

HEADACHE

Cold balm, basil, cayenne pepper, chamomile, ginger, marjoram, parsley, peppermint, rosemary, sage, garlic, lavender, valerian.

HEART

Asparagus, wild cherry, garlic, onions, hawthorn berries, lemon juice, valerian.

HEMORRHOIDS

Red potato, cocoa butter, witch hazel, yellow dock, bayberry, mullein.

HIGH OR LOW BLOOD PRESSURE

Yellow dock, garlic, ginger.

INFECTED SORES

Peach pits, garlic, cabbage juice.

INFLAMMATION

Comfrey, plantain, vinegar, witch hazel, garlic, cabbage juice.

ITCHING

Apple cider vinegar, anise, burdock, juniper, lemon juice, oat meal, yogurt.

JOINTS

Arnica, ginger, eucalyptus, olbas, onions, vinegar.

KIDNEY CONGESTION

Asparagus, cayenne pepper, parsley.

LAXATIVES

Fennel, licorice, psyllium, purslane, rhubarb, senna, sweet flag.

LIVER

Apples, beets, asparagus, burdock, caster oil, celery, centaury, chicory, coffee, dandelion, lemon juice, peppermint, prune, rosemary.

MEMORY

Asparagus, ginseng, gotu lola, rosemary, cabbage, bananas.

MENSTRUATION

Carrot, cayenne pepper, cinnamon bark, lemon juice, lentil, red raspberry, shepherd's purse, thyme.

MOUTH AND GUMS

Comfrey, goldenseal, myrrh, peach, oak bark, cabbage juice.

NAUSEA

Sweet basil, ginger, goldenseal, peppermint, black berry juice.

NEURALGIA

Allspice, celery, chamomile, coltsfoot, horseradish, juniper berries, lemon, peppermint.

NERVOUSNESS

Cumin, chamomile, clove, lavender, lime flowers, rosemary, valerian.

NIPPLES

Carrot, comfrey, yarrow.

NURSING (PROMOTE MILK)

Borage, dill, caraway, fennel, fenugreek, parsley, woodruff.

NURSING (STOP)

Sage.

POISON

Aloe vera, goldenseal, jewelweed, oat meal, vinegar.

RHEUMATIC PAINS

Parsley, juniper berries, cranberry juice.

SLEEP

Linden, chamomile, sage, catnip, clove skullcap, wormwood, lavender, balm.

SMOKING (Break the habit)

Chamomile, gentian.

SNAKE BITE

Rue, and see a doctor.

SORES

Goldenseal, myrrh, comfrey, lemon, honey, cabbage juice, garlic juice.

SPRAINS

Burdock, ginger, onion, garlic, vinegar.

SWIMMER'S EAR

Flush ear with equal amounts of alcohol and vinegar.

SWEATING HERBS

Yarrow, elder blossoms, chamomile, boneset, thyme, hyssop, catnip.

SWELLING

Comfrey, plantain, witch hazel, parsley, lavender, castor oil, carrot.

TONIC HERBS

Alfalfa, angelica, anise, basil, carrot, cayenne pepper, centaury, peppermint, raspberry, watercress.

VARICOSE VEINS

Cayenne pepper, marigold, oat bark, tansy, wood sorrel.

WARTS

Apple juice, cabbage, chickweed, dandelion, fig juice, houseleek, pineapple, watercress.

WORMS

Carrots, cayenne pepper, garlic, horseradish, lemon, pumpkin, tansy, thyme, wormwood.

GLOSSARY

A

ABORTIFACIENT - An agent which induces an abortion.
ACETYLCHOLINE - The substance which transmits cholinergic nerve impulses.
ADJUVANT - A substance which modifies the effect of another.
ALKALOIDS - A group of naturally occurring basic organic compounds which contains at least one nitrogen atom in a ring structure in the molecule. They are usually of plant origin, physiologically active, insoluble in water.
AMENORRHOEA - Absent of menstruation.
ANODYNE - A substance that relieves pain.
ANTIHELMINTIC - A substance which destroys or expels intestinal worms.
ANTI-MITOTIC - A substance which inhibits the division of cells.
ANTI-PYRETIC - A substance which prevents or reduces fever.
ANTI-SCORBUTIC - A substance which prevents of cures scurvy.
AROMATIC - (chem) Organic compound derived from benzene, also called aromatic compound; (herb) having fragrant and/or spicy taste or smell.
ASTHMA - Difficulty in breathing, due to constriction or spasm of air passages and caused by increased responsiveness of the bronchi and trachea to various stimuli, particularly allergy.
ASTRINGENT - A substance that causes contraction, shrinkage or firming of living tissues, often mucous membranes, and which is so doing reduces or stops the function of those tissues thereby effecting hemorrhages.
ATROPINE - An alkaloid obtained from members of the solanaceae family. It acts on smooth muscle and reduces secretions.

B

BILIOUS - Sometimes called Bilious. Either relating to the bile itself or to disorders caused by excessive production and release of bile into

the intestinal system.
BITTER- A substance characterized by a bitter taste. Often applied to alcoholic drinks containing bitter substances, or to botanical drugs with bitter constituents, which are used to promote the appetite.

C

CARMINATIVE - A substance which relieves flatulence and colic.
CATARRH - Excessive secretion from an inflamed mucous membrane, especially of the throat and head.
CATALYST - A substance which alters the rate at which a chemical reaction takes place, but itself remains unchanged at the end of the reaction.
CHOLAGOGUE - A substance stimulates or aids the release of bile from the gall-bladder.
CHOLERETIC - A substance which stimulates the production of bile in the liver.
COLIC - Acute paroxysmal pain in the abdominal region.
COUMARIN - A compound found in many plants and responsible for the aroma of new-mown hay which some possess. Ingestion in large amounts can lead to hemorrhage in man and animals.
COUNTER-IRRITANT - A substance that causes inflammation of the skin. It is applied for the temporary relief of a deep-seated painful irritation.
CYANOGENIC GLYCOSIDE - A glycoside which liberates hydrocyanic (or prussic) acid when broken down.
CYSTITIS - Inflammation of the bladder.

D

DECOCTION (herb) - Extract of a herb obtained by boiling a given weight of plant matter in a given volume of water for a given time.
DEMULCENT - A substance that is smooth and soothing when applied to an inflamed or painful surface.
DIAPHORETIC - A substance that causes an increase in perspiration. Some are used to treat fevers.
DIURETIC - A substance that increases the volume of urine and the frequency of urination.

DROPSY -An old-fashioned term for heart failure, characterized by the abnormal accumulation of serous fluid in body tissues.
DYSENTERY - Inflammation of the intestine, characterized by diarrhea containing mucus and blood, pain and painful straining to evacuate the bowels.
DYSPEPSIA - Disorder of the digestive process.

E

ECZEMA - An acute or chronic inflammatory disease of the skin of unknown causes.
EMETIC - A substance that causes vomiting.
EMMENAGOGUE - A substance that stimulates the menstrual flow.
EMOLLIENT - A substance used internally to soothe inflamed membranes, or externally to soften the skin.
ENEMA - The injection of fluid material into the rectum, usually for therapeutic purposes but occasionally to help diagnosis.
EPILEPSY - A brain disorder characterized by transient episodes or seizures during which convulsions and phychic dysfunction may occur.
ESSENTIAL OIL - A volatile oil, obtained from a plant by distillation and having a similar aroma to the plant itself.
EXPECTORANT - A substance which promotes the expulsion of fluid or semi-fluid matter from the lungs and air passages, by coughing or spitting.
EXTRACT - A product obtained by treating plant material with a solvent or mixture of solvents designed to extract the desired constituents.

F

FEBRIFUGE - A substance which prevents or reduces fever. Now known as anti-pyritic.
FIXED OIL - A non-volatile oil that cannot be distilled or evaporated without decomposition.
FLATULENCE - A condition in which excess gas is present in the

gastro-intestinal
FLAVONOID - A broad class of colored aromatic substances.

F

GALACTAGOGUE - A substance that can induce or increase the secretion of milk.
GALLIC ACID - An astringent substance.
GLUCOSIDE - A glycoside which yields glucose when broken down.
GLYCOSIDE - An organic substance which may be broken into two parts, one of which is always sugar.

H

HEMORRHAGE - Bleeding, the escape of blood from the blood vessels.
HEMOSTATIC - A substance that stops bleeding.
HALLUCINOGEN - A substance which can affect all or any of the senses, producing a wide range of perception and reaction.
HISTAMINE - Protective substance present in all tissues of the body, being released into the blood when, for example, the skin is cut or burned.
HYPOGLYCAEMIC - A substance that lowers the concentration of glucose in the blood.
HYPOTENSIVE - A substance that lowers the blood pressure

I

INFUSION - The preparation of a dose of a herb by pouring a given quantity of boiling water over a given weight of herb and infusion for a given time.
INGESTION - The act of taking in food or other material through the mouth.
INSULIN - A complex sugar found in several plants, especially in members of the family composite.

L

LACTATION - The secretion of milk.
LEACH - The extraction of soluble constituents from a mixture of soluble and insoluble material.
LEUCORRHEA -A white discharge from the vagina.
LINIMENT - A natural inorganic substance; often applied to the skin.

M

MACERATION - The process of extracting substances from a botanical drug by steeping in a solvent.
MENORRHAGIA - Excessive menstrual flow.
MINERAL - A natural inorganic substance; often applied to metallic salts and certain elements.
MOLLUSCIDAL - A substance that kill molluscs, such as snails.
MUCILAGE - A slimy product formed by the addition of gum to water. Mucilages occur naturally in many plants and may be applied to irritated or inflamed surfaces to relieve them.
MUCOUS COLITIS - Inflammation of the colon resulting in a mucous discharge.

N

NARCOTIC - A substance that in small doses produces sleep and relieves pain, but which in large doses may cause poisoning with coma or convulsions.
NERVINE (herb) - A substance that calms nervous excitement.
NEURALGIA - Brief but severe pain along the course of a nerve.

O

OXYTOCIC - An agent that hastens evacuation of the uterus by stimulating contractions.

P

PARASITICIDE - A substance that destroys parasites, especially those which exist on the skin.
PECTIN - A natural carbohydrate substance used as a demulcent or thickening agent.
PECTORAL - (med) Relating to the chest: (herb) a substance used in the treatment of chest complaints.
PHYTOTHERAPY - The medical use of plants, herbalists or medical herbalists.
POULTICE (herb) - Warm or hot external application of crushed herbs or extracts of plant contained in cloth.
PURGATIVE - A substance that causes evacuation of the bowels.

Q

QUINSY - Abscesses surrounding a tonsil.

R

RETARDANT (CHEM) - Serving to delay or slow down a chemical reaction.
RUBEFACIENT - A substance that causes reddening of the skin.
SAPONIN - A glycosidic substance that foams in water and has a detergent. Used as soap sometimes.
SCABIES - An infectious skin condition caused by a small insect.
SCROFULA - A tuberculous condition of the lymphatic glands, characterized by enlargement, suppurating abscesses, and cheese like degeneration.
SIALAGOGUE - A substance that initiates or increases salivation, the production of saliva.
SPASMOLYTIC - A substance that counteracts or relieves convulsions of spasmodic pains.
SPHAGNUM MOSS - A group of related mosses which grow in very wet places.
SPUTUM - Material eliminated from the mouth by spitting, consisting of secretions from the muscous membranes of the buccal cavity

which can include pus or blood.
STERNUTATORY - A substance that causes sneezing.
STOMACHIC - A substance that counteracts or relieves cramps.
STYPTIC - A substance that stops bleeding, usually by contracting the tissue.
SUDORIFIC - A substance that induces sweating.

T

TANNIN - Astringent substance related to tannic acid.
TINCTURE - A solution of substances extracted from medicinal plants by the maceration or percolation of the plant with alcohol or alcohol-water solution.

V

VASOCONSTRICTOR - A substance that causes the constriction of blood vessels.
VERMIFUGE - A substance that expels or destroys intestinal worms.
VOLATILE OIL - See essential oil.
VULNERARY - A substance used to treat or heal wounds.

COLLOQUIAL MEDICAL TERMS

ALL-OVERS - A nervous condition where nothing has gone right, and more is going wrong. About to blow your top.
TORRIABLY WELL - A person that is in good health, but doesn't want to admit it. - (Tolerably)
HOW YUH FEELN' - Say O.K. so I can tell you my complaints.
CONSUMPTION - A disease someone else has.

REFERENCE

Nearly all the herbal and folk medicine information presented in this book was compiled from records and oral interviews of herbal cures recorded by my parents for many years. Some of the information was handed down to them from their kin. Some of the information was brought here when their ancestors migrated over the many years from Montgomery County, North Carolina, then to Mayday area of Georgia, into Washington County, Alabama and Florida. Some went to Wayne, Simpson, Clark, Jasper, Perry County of Mississippi. Some went to Bald knob, Arkansas, then to the McCurtin County area of Oklahoma and De Queen, Arkansas. From this area to Texarkana, Texas, to Evans, Louisiana, and to Sabine Parish, Louisiana. All the families left Sabine Parish to many other areas. Some early families lived in Drew County, Desha, Union County, Arkansas and Monroe, Louisiana area. So this is why the herbal cures in this book is not limited to any one area.

My father collected herbs in the late twenties and most of the 1930's to sell. I started learning about herbs as soon as I was old enough to hold the sack for my father.

I have taken many oral interviews over the years from people who, by their age and background, would have knowledge of herbal and folk medicine. Most of these people have long since departed this world, and the information is lost forever with the exception of these interviews.

The following books may of help to you.

Brown, Claira, *Wild Flower of Louisiana,* LSU Press, Baton Rouge, Louisiana.

Price, Edward R. *Root Digging in the Appalachians.* The Bobbs-Merril, Los Angeles State College.

Watkins Cook Book. 1936, J. R. Watkins Co. Winona, Minnesota.

Altschul, S von Ries *Drugs and foods from little-Known plants* (Harvard University Press, Cambridge, Mass.

Burlage, H. M. *Index of plants with reputed Medicinal and Poisonous Properties* (Austin Press, Austin, TX 1968)

Poucher, W. A. *Perfumes, Cosmetics and Soaps* Volumes 1-3 (Chapman & Hall, London 1936)

Steward, F. C. *Plants at work* (Addison-Wesley, London 1964)

Swain, T. (ed) *Plants in the Development of Modern Medicine.* (Harvard University Press, Cambridge, Mass 1972)

HERBAL SOURCE

Penn Herb Co., Ltd, 603 North Street Philadelphia, PA 19123

Dried herbs, prepared herbal medicine, herbal oils, herbal candy, herbal juices, soaps, herbal deodorants, fragrant oils, seed for planting, books, and many other herbal items. Catalog $1.00

Rutland of Kentucky, P.O. BOX 16, Washington, KY, 41096

Herbal plants, seeds, oils, books, workshops and other herbal needs. Catalog $2.00

Caswell-Massey Co. Ltd., 76th Ninth Avenue, New York, NY 10011.

Dried herbs, fragrant oils, soaps, perfumes, herbal body powders, body oils and just about every herbal need. Catalog $1.00

Richters
Goodwood, Ontario
Canada LOC IAG

Herbal seed, dried herbs, books, essential oils, fixatives, spices, wildflower seed, herbal gardening supplies, and anything you would need in folk medicine.

THE TALKING HORNS

BLAM .... BLAM....... BLAM, It sounded across the quite countryside, most surely the sounds of a shotgun. All members of the household scampering out to the four sides of the house; waiting. BLAM......, another blast from a distant shotgun. The delayed shot was do the neighbors could get out and determine from where the shot came.) That shot would be about the Cook's place.

All strained their eyes in the direction of the cooks; looking for the tell tale glow flickering on the sky, a sure sign of a house fire. Nothing! No matter how hard they strained their eyes, nothing but the halo shadows of the early night. Grandpa Touch came from the house with his talkin' horn firmly grasped in his aging hands. You could see the flashes, from the now "lit" lantern, playing across the highly polished surface of the old cow horn. The horn was now honed and polished into a thing of beauty with a voice and tone of its own. No other horn would sound the same.

Grandpa Touch made his way up the creakily old latter to the roof of the house. Anyone could see Grandpa was getting old at ninety and four. He stood proud and erect, as well as his old frame would allow, bringing the horn to his mouth. He "rared" his head back, looking into the heavens, as if he were about to talk to his long since departed friends, the "talkin' horn gang." He let out a series of short blasts which echoed across the woodlands.

Again, he cupped his hand to his ears, waiting. In the distance came the sound of a up and down blast from another talkin' horn.

Grandpa Touch turned and yelled down in a wavering voice to the family on the ground. "Mr. Jones don't rightly know what are about at the Cook's. I will blow in Mr. Reyes and see if he knows."

Grandpa Touch again cupped his hand to his ears, listening to the other talking horns which were now sounding all around the countryside. "Clicky the click, the clop;" all could hear the sound of a horse coming at full speed down the lane which passed the house. Holding the lantern high, they could plainly see it was the Cook's boy on Old Lightning. He spoke not a word as he passed, which would indicate to the old-timers that this was a ride for life.

The only place the lane went was to Grandma Richardson's house, the local midwife and/or doctor for the area.

Grandpa Touch raised his talking horn and let out a blood curdling blast. All the talking horn went silent, as if Grandpa Touch was the switchboard of the horns. He turned in the direction of Grandma Richardson's and let out a long high pitched blast. Grandma Richardson could read the horns and would hitch up the buckboard and be on her way before the boy arrived.

Arriving at the Cook's, Grandma Richardson rushed into the dimly lit room as fast as her aging frame would allow. The only light was coming from the flickering fire in the fireplace. She could plainly see Grandma Cook was no more. She "fetched" a hot firecoal from the hearth of the old dirt chimney to make the test of death on Grandma Cook, Holding the firecoal with a pair of tongs, she touched it to Grandma Cook's arm and pitched the coal back into the fireplace. No blister! Grandma Cook was most' surely dead.

The low mournful wail of the talking horns could be heard all over the countryside, informing all within earshot that the code of death had begun for Grandma Cook. (A code of country protocol, which must be followed by all, the young and the old.)

(The title of Grandma or Grandpa didn't always denote kin. It was also a title of honor bestowed upon the old folks; most times, the oldest living member of each family clan.)

As Grandpa Touch's family neared the house of the cook's, the flicker of the fire, built out in the yard, lighted the sad faces of the men and children huddled around it in silence.

Grandma Cook was liked by all, the young and the aged. The wagon was tied to a tree near the yard, even now you could some women already entering the house wearing their old tattered and time-worn veils, some handed down from generation to generation, as times were very hard; but their pride was high, as pride was about all most of them had.

When the correct four women arrived (Protocol), they would dress out Grandma Cook in her Sunday's best. Grandma Cook's oldest kin would now, and only now, hand Grandma Richardson two old, time-worn coppers (large pennies) to place over Grandma Cook's eyes. (The dead were usually laid on boards, or a door placed on the bed. The coppers were kept in the family for kin only.) Now, the "sittin' with the dead must begin ."

The table in the side room kitchen had already several bowls of food on it brought by neighbors. They could ill-afford to bring this food such as it was; green, corn pones, a blackberry pie, some leftover chicken, and a bowl of boiled sow belly. (Food was never to be cooked in a house while sitting with the dead.)

The buryin' would be at sun's first light, the weather was warm and no one would wait until people could smell their kin.

Even now, out in the barn, some men were building a coffin from the sideboards of a neighbor's work wagon and several boards pulled from the walls of the old barn. (New lumber was not to be had at this late hour. Even if time permitted, there was no money, and it as a day's journey to the mill.)

Someone had already placed the cats in a chicken coop.

All the neighbors now started back to their homes to await the morning, with the exception of the women "sittin' up with the dead."

As the Touch's passed the graveyard, a short distance from the house, you could see the lanterns flickering as the bushes blocked their light when the wagon passed slowly by. There were just the ghostly shapes of some men digging the grave.

All of these things just seemed to happen without any direction from anyone as to who did what, in order to get ready for the buryin'. Maybe they had some custom that determined these things. "Never was able to find out for sure."

Grandpa Touch's family had settled in for the night, but only for a short moment, when the old roosters started their midnight crowing, bringing everyone to full 'wake. Back to sleep. No, not yet. In the distance came the roar of a mighty mallet pulling two hundred plus boxcars, flying through the night at full speed on the KCS Line. They say the engineer's name was Pynes, nobody knew for sure. He was blowing the saddest, most mournful, lonesome song ever "Blew" on a steam whistle. He roared on into the night 'til the sound faded, as if all the world knew Grandma Cook was dead.

After what seemed just a monent's sleep, the rooster started crowing for daylight. Everyone was up and out as the family chores had to be done fast, then to the buryin' at hand.

The old creaking wagon was hitched and the women folks climbed aboard with their "Sunday go meeting clothes" on, and those who had one, wore a black veil in place. Some stopped at the graveyard, some went on to the house. Everyone seemed to know where they should be. Even the people at "odds" with the Cook's were standin' quietly on a knoll some distance from the grave. To sit would show bad upbringin'. They, too, had a right to show the faces of their clan. This right was respected by all.

Out of the house came six men carrying the crude coffin, made with lumber that looked every day as old as Grandma Cook. Three mule belly bands were holding the coffin and the iron rings on each end of the bands were used as carrying handles. They set the coffin on a buckboard and started slowly to the grave site, "all the kin walking behind."

The little graveyard showed the sighs where someone had hoed and swept all the grass out with a freshly made dogwood broom which was, even now, leaning against a nearby tree. (To let the neighbors see grass in your graveyard was unthinkable and would cause the neighbors to gossip and think poorly of that family.)

A kindly neighbor with Bible learnin' started the final sayin's as the travelin' preacher, who preached in the brush arbor just down the road, would not be back 'til Sunday. He finished the sayin's, picked up a handful of lumpy clay and pitched it in the grave. Others did the same. Flowers? None, they would be planted at the next graveyard cleaning day.

No one noticed that Grandpa Touch and a few of the

older men were no longer at the gravesite. Two plow ropes were placed under the coffin, one at each end. four men lifted the coffin while the two cross-boards were removed by the other two men of the six.

As they started lowering the coffin into the ground across the graveyard came the most mournful, sad, spin-chilling sound ever to cross their ears. No one was in sight, but everyone knew it was form the men of the talkin' horns giving Grandma Cook a last farewell, and all knew they would not see the men for this day as they and their talkin' horns would just seem to fade away.

And, fade away they did--not just then, but not too many years thereafter. Were their deeds and time recorded in history? I don't think so, no recorded record of them has been located as of now. The coming of the T Model, A Model, radio and rural telephones was the beginning of the end of the talkin' horns.

I was told a few facts many years back by an old man pushing ninety. He said the horns were obtained from the Texas cattle drovers along the Nolan Trace. (The Nolan Trace is believed by many to be one of the four Texas-to-Louisiana cattle drover trails across Louisiana.) He further stated that his grandpa was used, along with other horn blowers, to keep General Walker's men informed of the where-abouts of the Yankees during the invasion of the Red River Valley. They could relay information to headquarters many miles away before a horse soldier could get started. Again, no record in the Official Records of the Civil War.) He stated that the horns were either "burnt" or buried with the horn blower, to insure that on one would ever attempt to blow a horn of the talkin' horn men.

Many of the "Old Timers" talked about the talking

horns but just couldn't remember much of what was said. Somewhere in a pack of old letters at the bottom of an old trunk, there may be some information on the talkin' horns; go look and see.

Even today, one old man claims if you listen long enough you will hear the sounds of the horns still floating across the hills and woodlands of Sabine Parish. I didn't have time to wait that long.

INDEX

C

D

E

F

G

H

I

W

Y